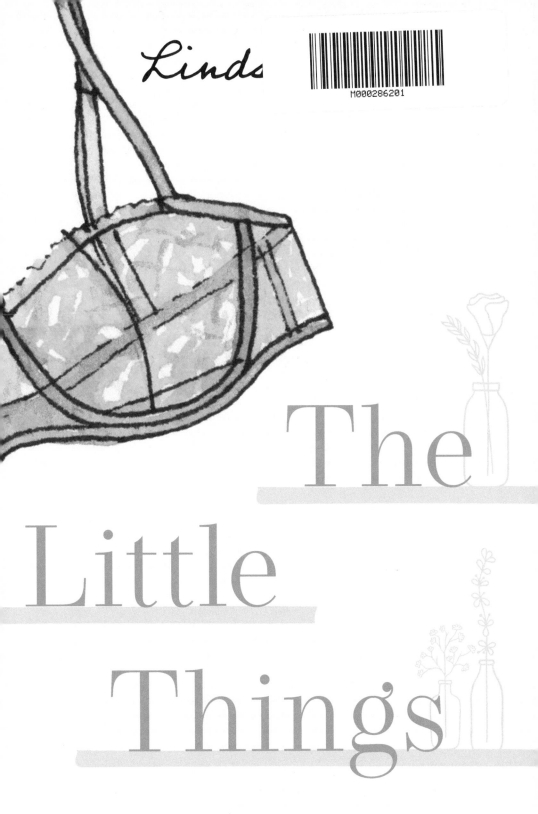

Linda

M000286201

The
Little
Things

A Breast Cancer Memoir

A catalogue record for this
work is available from the
National Library of Australia

Kennedy, Lindsey (author)
The Little Things: A breast cancer memoir
ISBN 978-1-922337-64-1
AUTOBIOGRAPHY

Typeset Font 11/15 Minion Pro

Edited by Vicki Englund
Author photo by Naomi Derrick Photography
My Breast Friends photo courtesy Nick Blair Photography
Cover and book design by Green Hill Publishing

*To my husband, John, who has loved and supported me
without complaint. Thank you. To my daughter, Layla,
thank you for always checking in on me. You continually
make me proud. Your smile is infectious and your strength
is remarkable. I love you. Master Lennox, thank you for
being a beautiful warrior. You make me laugh all the time
and I'm grateful for the special way you look after me.*

*To all my family and friends dotted all over the world
Thank you for your continued unconditional love and support.*

*To every care giver who gave me the best chance of
cancer never rearing its ugly head again, I thank you.*

*To Sean and Roisin, may we always fight
through our storms to get to our rainbows.*

*Be well
Lindsey
xx*

WARNING:

This book contains graphic images
that may offend some readers.

*You may need to download a QR reader on
your device to open suggested links on pages
77, 79, 81, 87, 94, 132, 162, 165 and 167.*

Contents

I heard it before I saw it, like someone turning on a tap, not quite a flow, but not a drip either. On the floor were large droplets of fluid, not blood, but not clear. I couldn't work it out, but I knew it was mine. I stiffened, delicately lifting my gown where I could see fluid leaking from my left breast. It had soaked through my breast dressing and was unapologetically rolling down the arc of my breast and down my stomach. I went through eight gowns over the next few hours. Each time I rose to move, it would ooze. It was sickening. A hematoma had burst inside my chest. For the next few weeks, I'd become very used to the same four hospital walls. The surgeries, chemotherapy and radiation had interrupted my life and my sleep, but what was to come would interrupt my physical being and try to bring me to my knees.

Introduction

In 2004, my younger brother, Sean, was diagnosed with non-Hodgkin lymphoma at nineteen years of age. While it devastated our family, he fought the battle of his life and won. Ten years later saw the breast cancer diagnosis of my only sister, Roisin (pronounced Ro-Sheen), who was pregnant at the time with her first child. With true grit, determination and the love of her family, she won her challenge.

Secondary cancer was an offensive, unwelcome visitor that violated Roisin yet again in early 2018. How dare it? How dare it invade again! Then my own visit to the doctor revealed a tiny 'speck' in my right breast. Unbelievably, I was given a positive diagnosis for breast cancer.

Writing this memoir came from an innate desire to make sense of what happened to me. By recording my events and thoughts, I wish to offer insight for others before, during and post-treatment for breast cancer. I want to provide hope for other cancer patients, their families and their friends.

Receiving a cancer diagnosis is life-changing. It can stop you in your tracks and halt time. These days, simply mention cancer, any cancer, and you realise that everyone knows someone who has it or who has had it. When it happened to me, it was an enormous shock and, sadly, all too familiar. It challenged my family's physical, psychological, spiritual and emotional wellbeing.

If you have been recently diagnosed, I'm not going to be so ignorant as to say it will be like this for you, but rather endeavour to record what my experiences were. We are all different; we all come in different shapes, ages and sizes. Each person's cancer journey is different, but, with breast cancer, there are similarities. Not everybody diagnosed will experience the same type of cancer, have the same kind of treatment nor the same level of care as myself, because our stories are all individual.

There are hundreds and thousands of experiences out there, but this one is unique to me. I wrote this book as I observed a high-interest level about breast cancer among my friends and my community. I figured penning my journey could help others understand the logistics and the nitty-gritty, and provide a 'dummies guide to' – a behind-the-scenes look at an individual's grapple with breast cancer.

I am not a medical professional of any kind. I'm offering a brief look into my very personal experiences that you may or may not find useful. I'm not telling anyone how to deal with their experience, as we all have different paths to walk and individual decisions to make. It has not been a journey for me; it has been one long pilgrimage. I intend to weave some of my private stories into my writing in order to be raw and honest about what happened to me.

I have written in the truest way I can. I have allowed myself to write about my vulnerabilities, holding the mantra in my head: *Telling my story may help somebody navigate theirs.* Writing has been incredibly cathartic for me and happiness has never been too far away when I've relived some of my memories over the past few years. I can emphatically say I enjoyed writing this book as it reminded me to focus on the simple things, not to rush life and to slow down and smell those damn roses!

I came to the stark realisation that without intervention, my own body would have killed me. What the hell was my flesh and blood doing working against me? In the end, I've learned that maybe everything I went through was trying to build me, not break me.

> *'It's a bloody cruel old tosser, cancer. Lindsey, Sean and*
> *I are so lucky to be here to enjoy the smallest of things,*
> *today – right now – because, really, that's all we have.'*
> Roisin Pelan

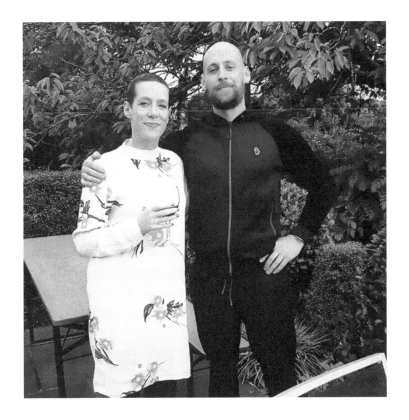

Roisin and Sean celebrating the end of her radiation therapy. 2019.

One

The history of us

*'Write it on your heart that every day is the best day in the
year. He is rich who owns the day, and no one owns the
day, who allows it to be invaded with fret and anxiety.'*
Poet, Ralph Waldo Emerson

I simply adored my childhood.

Born and raised a Lancashire lass in the northwest of England meant that I always had many street friends. It was a childhood where, if your mum wasn't around, someone else's mum could step up to the job and fix anything: a bump, a scrape or even a sandwich if needed. One of six children, I was the second eldest and the firstborn daughter. Growing up, our street was one big happy family. Like so many childhoods before mine, rope swings were a favourite pastime. Endless hours were spent swinging and spinning around, until one day, one of the neighbourhood kids hit his head so hard on the tree trunk that the 'ropey' reached its demise and had to be cut down. When I close my eyes, I can still hear the *thump* of that boy's poor crown.

We played outdoors throughout all seasons – unaccompanied of course – only navigating our way home for four reasons: a toilet stop, a drink, food, or because we were beckoned by our parents as the street lights flickered, indicating our day's play was over. We had fierce games of football (soccer) between families that would last for weeks and we got filthy, absolutely filthy. God knows how much mud and soil we ingested as children, but it was regarded as feeding our immune systems and a belief that this was why we barely missed any school. Like a conch from the South Pacific, our parents called us in by opening the front door and shouting our names from eldest to youngest in the hope that they would hear our twelve thunderous, competitive footsteps. Indoors, we would settle into our evenings watching classic shows such as *Blue Peter*, *Swap Shop* and *Tizwas* on the TV.

My mum, Margaret, is one in a million. She is an eccentrically hilarious drama queen and there is never a dull moment in her company. We were not together enough during my younger years because she held down two jobs and worked night shifts. There were many days where we didn't even cross paths. Even without her physical presence in the house, she was someone I shared my deepest secrets with and the person on whom I could always count. She taught me the joys of black and white film, craft, books, and I attest my solid work ethic to simply being her daughter.

My dad, Tony, is a gentle giant. His soft Belfast accent never fails to draw you in. I adore him. Growing up, I was obsessed with him and still am now if I'm honest. He used to do my hair for school and make us all delicious hot toast for supper. My dad was the dad that took us all out to discover every

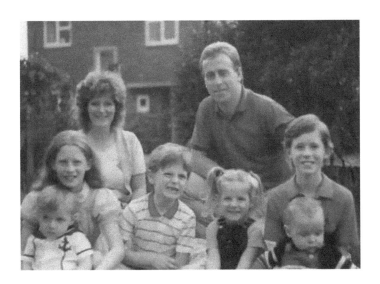

Summer of 1985, here I am, aged eleven, holding my brother Michael. I love Mum's perm in this picture!

possible mountainside trek or winding canal known to man. He is my hero. Growing up in a small three-bedroomed house, adventures were staples and prevented us all from going stir-crazy. Mum and Dad both stepped up when I needed them most and I will always cherish that time together forever. Even now, in an attempt to feel close to my parents or to appease feeling homesick, I gravitate to my bedside table which is stuffed with personal trinkets from my life in the U.K.

Aged nineteen and meeting my Australian now-husband, John, in England in August of 1993 was one of life's great moments. We met in a busy club where a mutual friend introduced us. I was smitten from the moment I met him. He was a diminutive seventeen year-old soccer-playing ball of muscle with a strong Australian accent and a tanned complexion. He had a huge smile and I was intent that night that he'd win my phone number. Cheeky, but it worked!

In my second year of university, I moved into student accommodation, renting a house with five others. With a room that mimicked my childhood home, it housed a bed, desk, wardrobe and other student basics. John had moved from Australia and had been living in Preston for a year when we met. So began our love affair.

Four years later having gained a degree and a teaching certificate, I migrated to Australia in July 1997. I was twenty-three and had never been on an aeroplane. I often chuckle to myself, *Why did I have to meet an Australian, of all people?* Sporting the whitest skin known to humanity and millions of freckles, I literally crisp up in any weather over fifteen degrees. I have an English/Irish background that has forced me over the past twenty or so years to sit in the shade with factor-50 lathered on and armed with a good book. I've probably singlehandedly prevented many a sunscreen company from financial collapse.

Missing my family while living in Australia was standard. Materialistically, we didn't have a lot growing up, but we were showered with love and were always open and honest with each other. Mum taught us to be strong and outspoken while Dad taught us to appreciate each other's differences and how to love unconditionally. We were well connected then and still are to this day.

Not long after my emigration, I gained my first teaching position at a school I loved. I made friends quickly and settled into Aussie life easily. John and I were married in 2004 on a stunning beach in Mount Eliza, Victoria. We were blessed with a perfect ceremony followed by a winery reception which topped off what had been a fantastic decade of fun and adventure. We honeymooned in Thailand and planned to take off for a year to England where we could reconnect with our English families and travel around Europe at the same time.

Everything seemed so wonderful, but there were dark clouds gathering around my youngest brother, Sean. He has been a source of hilarity since the day he was born. Many a fond memory of him and the role he played in our family still makes me laugh out loud to this day (If we ever meet, ask me about the pickle story). We teased Sean all the time for upsetting the rhythm of babies being born. Until he arrived, it had been boy, girl, boy, girl, boy... and then Sean! Then, when he grew the roundest, cutest, curly blonde afro, we all felt justified to continue with our taunts. I'm not ashamed to say he was my favourite. He has piercing blue eyes and a vivacious personality that just made us all so happy. I even used to pretend that I was his mum at the young age of eleven. Watching Sean go through a cancer diagnosis as a teenager and truly fight for his life was just heartbreaking, and on the crappy days when I think about cancer too deeply, it still is.

While in England, a dinner invitation with Sean marked the beginning of a massive family upset. He was just a teenager. While we were eating and chatting, I noticed that he had his head cocked to one side and I *don't* think it was because he was intently listening to me blabber on. I quizzed him and he explained that it had been like that for a while and that he was struggling a bit at work and the gym. When he left, I immediately rang Mum to express my concern. Mum told me that both she and Dad had known in their hearts that Sean had been unwell for months but that he simply was taking his time to go to the doctor. In a bid to protest his ignorance, she had once gone on a hunger strike, but lasted two days as she got peckish (told you she was eccentric!).

Sean had symptoms, but was reassured by a doctor that all was well. As a young person, he chose to not worry and just get on with life – a behaviour

I've seen before. Ill-health, of course, *should not* be ignored, and to Mum, he was just being stupid! He was really unwell at this point. He was short of breath, white as a ghost and I knew he was just putting on a brave face. A biopsy revealed a huge mass in his neck, leading to a diagnosis of non-Hodgkin lymphoma. We were devastated. As a family, it rocked us to the absolute core.

I believe that my being in England at this turbulent time and able to be part of the journey that Sean was to travel, was the work of angels. I resigned from my ongoing school contract and John and I agreed that we'd stay in the U.K. until a doctor told Sean that he was N.E.D. (no evidence of disease). He fought HARD, and we helped support him through the toughest fight of his life. After his last radiation therapy session, we all met in the hospital car park with a bottle of champagne. We smiled and cheered and filled our day with love for Sean. When we arrived home, we all had a crazy marshmallow fight in the dining area as a manic release of stress. Looking back on these photos makes me smile, thinking of how brave he was.

These days, Sean lives in Bradford, England with his partner, Mary. He did have a skin cancer diagnosis in December 2019, but it was localised and everyone involved is confident that it is all gone. He is a personal trainer too, a job at which he's a natural.

Sean's recovery took the best part of two years. John and I left, bound for Australia in September 2006.

SEAN:

'When something happens to your family, you feel it deep in your heart, whether it's the announcement of a new baby, a wedding, passing your driving test or someone falling ill. Unfortunately, the last one was lurking in our family, and not just for one of us. At the end of my last year in school, and as early as sixteen years old, I felt different, but I left it and put it down to my transitioning from boyhood into a hulk of a man.

Moving forward, I had good health days and unusual health days. I was concerned and so were my parents. Frustrated, I requested a new G.P. who took one look at me and I could see he had worries. I went for an immediate biopsy on a lymph gland at the hospital and the dreaded wait at home followed. My parents walked into my bedroom, both teary and frozen to the spot. My mum kept repeating, "It's good news, it's good news. They can cure it." I had been diagnosed with stage three non-Hodgkin lymphoma. I beat cancer and all with a smile, but don't be fooled – it was life-changing, devastating and at times crippling. It was hard, and I certainly had bad days, but I fought it for my family. So that's it. Our bad luck was out of the way...'

We were to have a quiet decade. It was now that John and I realised it was time to tackle some 'grown-up' behaviours, so we purchased a small weatherboard house at the 'Paris end of the Peninsula' in Frankston – a suburb of Melbourne, Victoria. It was built in 1954 not far from the beach. We moved in when I was eight months' pregnant with our first child, Layla. Our son, Lennox, was born two years later and we decided that our baby-making was complete. We settled into a comfortable life filled with friends, family, renovations, travel and adventure.

Once again, bad news wasn't far away. May 2014 brought a phone call revealing my sister's first cancer diagnosis. Roisin skyped us to tell us the news and it was just awful.

A little bit about my sister – she arrived in 1981 and at the age of eight, I found myself in seventh heaven! A sister, a girl, for me, to keep, forever. She is so amazing and growing up with her was a pleasure. We shared a small bedroom. Once a set of bunk beds, a wardrobe and a dresser were in it, there was no room for dancing.

Growing up, Roisin was a sensitive girl and I would try my best to comfort her in the mornings. She would always cry about the same two things – one was the fear of being late for school, which we never were, and the other was separation anxiety. She never wanted to leave our parents, ever. Even now, as an adult, she lives a mere four-minute drive away from them, the total opposite of me. As the sister of an unwell sibling, it brings me peace that, no matter what, our parents are there for her, always.

Back to that terrible phone call. Roisin appeared on the screen with her partner, Michael Brown, (we have to call him that due to one of my brothers being named Michael). She was in the late stages of pregnancy. 'I have something to tell you and I don't want you to cry', she said, managing a nervous smile. Even as the words fell... 'lump'... 'cancer'... my shoulders squared and an overpowering, protective sense of what it was I had to do swept over me.

Feeling angry, I was off to war. I was determined it would be a war we were going to win. Never was there a doubt in my mind that her cancer was going to be weaker than we were. I thought we'd been through enough after Sean. We had beaten cancer once as a family, so we knew we could do it again! We all held optimistic mindsets from the start. There was just no other way to think. But I still found myself scratching my head, searching for answers.

Panic saw me book a ticket back to England the very next day. John took some of his long- service leave to play single dad as our children were only six and four at the time – a selfless act that made me love him even more. Shortly after, I made the familiar trip home to offer help in any way I could. Mum herself had developed ill-health not long after Sean's diagnosis. I was battling with a sick mother, sick brother, a sick sister and was left wondering, where had we gone wrong? Was it our fault? Did we have a dodgy family gene? Was it our diet? Was it living near huge pylons with high-voltage electricity pulsing through them? So many unanswered questions. I just didn't know how to process my thoughts.

Not long after Roisin's diagnosis, she prematurely gave birth to a beautiful, baby girl, Ivy. A few days later, she had a single mastectomy and not long after that started chemotherapy. Everything happened so fast, leaving me desperate to embrace her and tell her I loved her. In an instant, she had lost her breast, her hair, her confidence and the maternity leave of which she had been dreaming.

I had made this long-haul trip across the globe many times before. I was greeted at Manchester Airport by my parents and a very excited Roisin and Michael Brown holding my tiny five-week-old niece. The reunion was marred a little with sadness, but this was soon overshadowed when I held that little ginger-haired baby. I was in love. She was perfect and I knew I was going to do my best to look after her, hoping that would give Michael and Roisin some quality time together. What a roller coaster it had been for them so far – a cancer diagnosis, their first baby, a single mastectomy and Roisin starting on chemotherapy! It all seemed surreal.

They had a beautiful house, full of colour, vibrancy and bunting – Roisin loves bunting. She buys it or makes it and it follows her everywhere like a loyal friend. In my room, there was a huge, framed poster reading '*Welcome home Lindsey*' and I loved it. (Even though I reside in Australia, I still call England my home – a permanent bone of contention between John and me.)

Their house was never silent. Michael Brown is a musician, specialising in the drums, and music is on from dusk till dawn, which is both uplifting and relaxing. Throughout my stay, tending to Ivy was a privilege that I treasured every day. Feeding her, snuggling with her, even changing her nappy transported me back to happy times with our young children. Whether she felt it or not, I had made a strong bond on that trip and I knew leaving her would be terribly difficult.

Ironically, Roisin worked part-time in the office of the oncology department at her local hospital. I accompanied her to one of her chemotherapy sessions during my trip. She was part of the system already; she was the front face you saw upon arrival for chemotherapy sessions. What a person to be greeted by! Naturally smiley, warm and empathetic, no doubt she would have appeased people there for the first time, filled with worry and stress, by giving them her full attention.

We walked through to her appointment and she was greeted by all who passed her. I observed the ghastly process as her chemotherapy began. Carefully and clinically, pillar box red poison was intermittently injected into her veins. My heart thumped against my rib cage. I was emotional. I tried to hide it, but my heart ached. We tried to mask it by having a laugh, cracking chemo jokes (a sense of humour is always required) and generally being goofy, but inside, the reality of my beautiful baby sister being pumped with poison was horrific to me. Knowing I had only a few precious weeks with her made it even harder. What I didn't know then was, just four short years later, *I* would be the one sitting in a chemotherapy chair.

As a teenager, I moved out of home to attend university. Missing my sister lasted for a very long time. She has gone on to build a solid relationship with her man, Michael Brown. Together, they have Ivy, an intelligent six year-old at the time of writing this, and the adorable Master Teddy, a little chubby cherub who never stops smiling. My sister builds positive relationships with everyone close to her. She is one of those people that you are drawn to; you can't help it. She's very charismatic and someone you don't forget in a hurry. When thinking of my relationship with her, I compare it to the ancient concept of yin and yang. We are opposite in many ways, but have a splash of each other within ourselves. We also have a great sense of how our personalities complement each other. We laugh when we're together and always hold each other in high regard.

During my time in England, I caught up with many family members and long-time friends. As always, it was a whirlwind trip but I'm so glad I did it. Leaving was ridiculously hard – I was torn in two. I knew that the rest of my life was in Australia, but I longed to live back home so much and it wasn't the first time I would feel this way.

When I was a teenager, Roisin bought me a bottle of Sunflowers perfume, which I loved. I would spray it on my pillow to remind me of her. We promised each other that we would sign off our text messages with a sunflower emoji to be forever connected. She then added that I could have the sunflower, but she wanted a lightning bolt and a rainbow because she was determined to weather the storm and come out of this shining like a rainbow. That was lovely, but if she was having two, I wanted two! My heart was set on a strong-arm emoji to represent how tough we were both going to be. Doing this that night helped me manage my emotions, and landing back on Aussie soil, I had a sense of being brave, strong and all-round hardcore.

Two

The big squeeze

'It's about taking the traumatic moments in life that are scattered around us and sewing them back together into something beautiful that maybe emboldens people who are going through the same thing – which we all are because the 'same thing' is life, and it's hard and screwed up but delicious.'
Ariel Gore

One hot morning in the Australian summer holidays of January 2018, I awoke to the familiar sound of an overseas ringtone on my phone. It was my sister. After a swift glance at the clock, I noticed it was very early, which was unusual. I generally heard from Roisin in the evening because of the time difference. Moving to the lounge room, I tiptoed as the house slept. My usual cheery outlook turned sour very quickly as she was calling to tell me that she had been re-diagnosed with stage 3C breast cancer. It turned into what I *thought* was the worst day of my life.

When Roisin told me she had cancer the second time, something left me. The words, 'It's back' choked me. No, they strangled me. I was paralysed by fear. I wasn't informed enough. What on earth?? She had no breasts, what was going on? I'm embarrassed to admit that I thought if cancer ever came back, most of the time you died. I was rendered speechless.

Things happen at the speed of light when you receive bad news. Multiple things to say raced through my mind, but I found myself crying and powerless to speak. Roisin was repeatedly apologising and my stomach somersaulted in pain. John jumped up out of bed to see what was going on and, pushing the phone to his chest, I sobbed. I just couldn't pull myself together there and then. Asking her to give me ten minutes to make a cuppa and to sort myself out would afford me the time to wander down to the back of the garden and scream into my hands.

Being overwhelmed like that was something that had never happened before in my life. I was briefly frantic. Gathering my thoughts as I inhaled the hot brew of camomile tea, my fingers trembled as I dialled. John was with me as we heard how Roisin had found a lump in her neck and things had gone bad from there. We heard how she had to push for scans as she found herself being offered suggestions by health professionals as to what it could be. These suggestions were reasonable, but she was convinced that they were wrong – one hundred per cent wrong. Finishing that phone call left me broken-hearted.

After quickly contacting my school principal, who was overseas at the time, and receiving the go-ahead for three weeks off, I booked flights that very day, just like last time. This time, all four of us were going to England for Easter. Duty called.

Sleeping was a struggle for the next few days. I could hear the soft, sad tones of my sister, my baby thirty-six year-old sister, giving me the bad news. It tormented my mind. Her words, when I let them, still haunt me.

Given the circumstances, my local G.P. suggested a thorough check-up. He'd only been my doctor a little over two years, but we've always been very trusting of one another. He clearly explains things to me and I feel like I work well with him to make comprehensive medical decisions.

Having a good doctor is vital. Many people admit to me that they don't change doctors, even if they don't necessarily like them, or get the outcome they want, or if they disagree with what they suggest because 'He has been my family doctor for years', or 'They'll do, I don't go to the doctors often anyway'. Loyalty is admirable, but not at the expense of your future health. It is really important to feel respected and understood by your G.P. You also need to be able to say the embarrassing (to some) words such as breasts, nipples and vagina, even if it means squirming in your seat. If this is not the case, my advice would be – you NEED to change doctors.

This can be challenging, but if there is one thing I've learned about my journey it's that self-advocacy is paramount when dealing with this dreaded disease. BCNA **www.bcna.org.au** (Breast Cancer Network Australia), established in 1997, is an organisation that positively influences the way breast cancer is considered in the community and they can help support you with this transition if required. It seems strange to think a doctor could be bad for our health, but in some circumstances, they can.

So, the thorough check-up began. A previous ultrasound eight months earlier left me feeling at ease. The report came back normal and, like so many times before, I was unphased. A check of my breasts by hand revealed nothing to worry about, offering me instant relief. My G.P. then suggested some diagnostic testing, a mammogram and an ultrasound back-to-back on the same day. Under normal circumstances, I would have had one or the other.

It was a Wednesday and I was four days away from returning to my teaching position and starting my twenty-first year of teaching. I booked an appointment at the local radiologists for my mammogram and ultrasound, but found that the earliest appointment was a month later. I reluctantly accepted. My mind raced when I arrived home and the need to seek an earlier appointment nagged me. My sister had been re-diagnosed and I deemed it unacceptable at this point for me to wait that long. I managed to find a morning appointment the day before Australia Day, January 25th. Thankfully, my sister-in-law Ginny, visiting from Brisbane, was free to look after our children. Layla was now ten and an extraordinary acrobat with a zest for life, and Lennox, an energetic, soccer-playing eight year-old. I left John sleeping and made my way to the life-altering appointment.

Mammograms, or as I prefer, 'the big squeeze', can be free for eligible women. A screening program through BreastScreen Victoria in Australia, for whom I'm a proud ambassador, offers free breast screens for asymptomatic women (no symptoms). These target women between the ages of 50 – 74 biannually. This organisation aims to reduce the impact of a breast cancer diagnosis and ensures the best health outcome through early detection.

Funded by the Victorian and the Commonwealth Governments, the procedure takes ten minutes, is always with a female radiographer and no doctor's referral is needed. It is during this screening that four x-rays of your breasts are taken and reviewed by radiologists. These films are kept and referred to at your next appointment two years later, when the radiologists look for any changes.

At my appointment, I was taken into the room which housed the mammogram machine (x-ray machine). Very slowly, my breasts were sandwiched between two plates (paddles) and the images taken. It was not a new experience for me, but this time I felt pain. Screwing up my eyes and inflating my lungs allowed me to tap into my yoga breathing. Inhale for six, hold for two and exhale for six. It didn't take long before hearing the standard statement, 'Remain in your gown. We will check the films and be back shortly.'

Trying to not get caught taking mammogram selfies was how I used the wait time. Being a forty-four year-old woman and getting caught taking selfies would have been a bit embarrassing, given my situation! It remains odd to me that I looked and felt so good on this day, yet something was about to be tracked down and pulled out of hiding. Uploading a selfie on my socials, titling it, **'check your boobs, people'** was in support of my sister. It was also to awaken the beast in me to encourage other people to check their breasts – an action that we cannot afford to shy away from.

I became aware that the mammographer was taking a little longer than usual but thought nothing of it. I had noticed the waiting room was full and there was no doubt that my films were probably in a queue. Or were they? My mind started to race and a tiny pang of worry catapulted in my brain. I thought of my two beautiful nannas who'd fought cancer twice, my kid brother and now my sister, also twice. I had, in a five-second window, totally convinced myself that I was in some sort of trouble. The pendulum began to swing. Who was I kidding? I lived in the land of plenty, one of the most liveable cities in the world. All will be well. Cancer wasn't ever going to get me. But what if? My self-talk went into overdrive. *No, you're just being silly.*

This went on for what seemed an eternity and my heart raced and thumped until the nurse returned and stated, 'All good. Just pop next door for your scheduled ultrasound', as she rushed off to get the next 'big squeeze' patient in line. *Phew*, I told myself. Of course, they were busy. I had myself half-convinced.

I was led into a darkened room for my breast ultrasound. The technician was a young male and I recognised him from previous ultrasounds – I'd become an 'over-checker' after my sister's first diagnosis. We exchanged a few niceties as he placed a wedge pillow under my shoulder blade, making my breast look somewhat like an oversized fried egg. He then squirted cold gel over the probe. I was once fortunate enough to experience an ultrasound using a pre-warmed gel and I tell you, it was a game-changer.

He began the hunt in my right armpit. He didn't get far before hovering there for a little bit too long for my liking. Had he started there because of the mammogram result? He continued the search on that breast for ages. I stayed unusually silent, listening, aware only of my increasing heartbeat. Normally, I would have asked if something had been found or if I had anything to worry about. This time, on this day I didn't, and I still don't know why. I couldn't speak and had a serious case of lockjaw – the calm before the storm maybe? He checked my left breast with equal caution, then, placing a small white towel over me, he left the room. I recall thinking that if he came back with a second person, *I have cancer*. It was that simple to me.

Minutes later, he walked in with a breast surgeon.

Topless, with only a small towel over my chest, a huge breath left me. I calmed myself by playing the distraction game, complimenting the surgeon on her dress. I was aware I was doing this, perhaps wanting to lighten the mood in the room as I knew it was about to turn dark. My mind raced. She warmly introduced herself and took my hand in hers. I'm so grateful she did this. Did she know my history? Did she know about Sean and Roisin? She made me aware that something had come up on the ultrasound that looked sinister and that my doctor had been contacted. Wait, she had contacted my doctor? What?! Knowing this freaked me out. It was real now.

She then said not to worry because it was only small. I knew that when an ultrasound was done it was with high-frequency sound waves. The sound waves echo differently when they bounce off something irregular. Those waves had just crashed all over my chest and my life was to be irreversibly changed.

Lying down, I felt powerless, vulnerable and out of control, but sitting up led to a burning sensation filling my throat and nervous energy lining my veins. I hadn't brought anyone with me because it was never going to happen to me, remember? Tears stained my cheeks and I felt the muscles of my chin spasm like an anxious child. I shared with them that I couldn't have anything wrong with me because I'd booked a flight to England to nurse my unwell sister. Roisin needed me because *she* had cancer. It dawned on me then that I needed to ask if *I* actually had cancer. This was sidestepped with the standard retort of, 'Pathology will determine that', which was fair. *Yes*, I thought, *it will determine that I am positive for cancer.*

Not realising I was crying, I was handed a box of tissues by the young man who had performed the ultrasound. He touched my shoulder, instantly calming me. It was suggested John meet me at the doctor's rooms and I left with a heavy heart and red eyes. It was on the drive home that I lost the ability to stop crying, my mind was tangled and my hands were shaky. I had to pull over at one point to compose myself. I knew I was sick. I lost count of how many questions I asked myself in that five-minute break.

Calling John, I was convinced that I had pulled myself together. I hadn't. As the phone was ringing I used self-talk to prepare, but that didn't work. I cried my eyes out when he answered, and once again those very recognisable words 'lump' and 'cancer' fell from my lips. Even without pathology results, I knew this was not a good situation.

When I met John, I could see that he'd been crying. Cradling his face and wiping away his tears, I reassuringly told him that everything was going to be okay and that no way on God's green earth was I going to die from this. We went in holding hands but not talking. When my G.P. saw me, he beckoned us into his consulting room with an oversized wave in the air that ended wrapped around my shoulders. *He knows*, I thought.

Let me say here that I'm so incredibly fond of my corduroy-wearing, gum-chewing Polish doctor. We continue to make a good team and he keeps me on the right side of sane. Again, I was told that pathology was the only way to diagnose me and he contacted a breast surgeon with whom I had dealt a few years earlier. She was young, to the point and I liked her. I scheduled the first available appointment, which was four days after the initial find. Everything was closed on Australia Day... then it was Saturday... then it was Sunday and time seemed to stand still. I managed to be the surgeon's first Monday morning appointment.

Upon waking, butterflies raced like cyclists in a velodrome inside my stomach because I'd talked myself into my breast surgeon announcing that I had cancer as soon as I crossed her office threshold. In the car on the way, Macklemore came on the radio and, the lyrics, 'Someday soon, your whole life's gonna change', sent a tingle down my spine. My surgeon had reviewed the reports and wasn't sure if it was or wasn't cancer. A glimmer of hope teased me. She was on the fence and I was on a high. Half of me was jumping for joy, kicking up my heels, while the other half was in a corner sucking my thumb. It was a weird paradox to be in and one that I didn't wish upon anyone.

The next day, I had to attend a citizenship ceremony of one of my closest friends, Mandy. I hope she knows how welcome a distraction that was. Wearing bright lipstick, I wore my 'fake it till you make it' face and got through the day, but on the inside I was really worried. I had developed a very strange unfamiliar sensation. It was as though my upper arms had locked. They were very tense and I struggled to use them. My doctor suggested to me later that it was probably fear. I can still recall that feeling now and again, like a bad memory, but in a physical sense. Throughout that weekend, I had a serious case of the jitters.

My breast surgeon organised for me to have a biopsy of the lump. She advised bringing someone with me as I was going to be slightly sedated. I planned to, without a doubt, that person being my sister-in-law, Ginny. I had learned the hard way the power of a support partner from my experience days earlier. Feeling blue getting ready for the appointment, I realised it was supposed to be the first day for me starting back as a full-time teacher. How my life had changed.

During my biopsy, I couldn't have asked for better nurses. They were bursting with concern, understood my anxiety, and I could feel they were on my side. I was given a sedative followed by a local anaesthetic in my right breast. A small incision was made and a straw-type device placed into my breast, all under the guidance of an ultrasound. Another thinner instrument was placed down the straw-shaped device, taking samples of the tumour. It sounded like the click of an EpiPen and was slightly uncomfortable. I was told by the doctor that my lump was 'a toughie'. Yuk! The doctor was quietly spoken and another glimmer of hope shot my way. He believed it looked like a fibroadenoma, which is a non-cancerous breast lump. I didn't get too excited. I think I still just knew and was silently crying hot tears. (As I've said, the two wonderful nurses were onto this very quickly.) I left with a small bandage, and Ginny and I agreed no one should be worried until we got the results.

It was a Tuesday and had been six days since the lump was discovered. Even without the results, I began to rehearse what I'd say when I looked down the camera to tell my parents, family and most of all, my beautiful sister, that I too was sick. The brain is a wonderful thing. Each time I reached the point in my thoughts where family members appeared on my phone screen, my brain drew a line in the sand and stopped me from staging that scenario. I was booked in to get my results late afternoon on Friday. Three sleeps to go…

The next day, John and I had to have a serious conversation. Earlier in the year, he had been asked to travel to Queensland for three weeks' work. John is a carpenter by trade and had been working hard as a leading hand, in order to be recognised and considered for future promotion. I thought it was a good choice for him to go and he promised he would video-call every day. It was all set. Twenty-four years together and he has never had to work away. The timing had the potential to be disastrous. The flights were booked for Friday – results day – but John rearranged them for the Saturday so he could be with me either to celebrate or console me.

The next day, my Homey, Naomi, came over. Naomi is one of those friends who just gets it. She knows when to say and do the right thing at the right time. She turned up with a bunch of sunflowers, a vivacious three year-old and a massive smile. We chatted the afternoon away and the distraction was welcome. The scent of the sunflowers formed many happy memories for me and this flower became symbolic in my life. A sunflower is tall and strong and they are known to be happy flowers. They symbolise longevity too, a sentiment I was gripping onto at this tense time.

I spent Thursday with Cindy, my closest friend. She became intimately involved in my health and wellbeing from the get-go, and has become my sister and counsellor all rolled into one. Her personality type means people from all walks of life are interested in her. I met her through her brother, Damo, in a mutual place of work in 1999. After two weeks of knowing him, he suggested I meet his sister. We became close very quickly. Migrating to Australia with only a boyfriend and a backpack, I soon found myself adopted into their large Mauritian family. Cindy would turn up in her leisurewear and lip gloss most Thursdays and we would eat and chat the afternoons away. This day, however, without her realising it, Cindy became my distraction. My anxiety was high. It was the eve of results day and I knew John was about to leave the following day regardless. Ginny stepped in and gave me words of comfort and warmth. She always has a fabulous sense of humour, which I really needed at this time. However, I was still fairly scared out of my wits.

Later that evening I decided to video-call my parents to let them know what was going on. I was in that 'calm before the storm' frame of mind again. As I said the word 'lump', once again I froze. No words came out – I willed myself to talk, but no words emerged. I was covering my mouth and weeping. Explaining through tears that I was really worried, I apologised over and over to them for potentially being the third of their children to maybe have cancer. A bit dramatic I know, but I wasn't in control here; my emotions were all over the place. My parents calmed me down and after a long chat laced with reassurance, I turned off the video-call, exhausted.

Three

Dealing with diagnosis

*'Some things just happen and we
don't ever get to know why.'*
Melissa Sotelo

I now realise that nothing could have stopped me from getting cancer, no matter how many vegetables I ate, no matter how much sugar I cut out, no matter how many squats or lunges I managed, no matter *what* I did. Cancer did not respect me as a person. It just invited itself in, set up camp and wreaked havoc… that is, until it was caught.

We were all so busy living our lives, then all of a sudden, something powerful cut through our routine – something life-changing. John stopped me on the way into the clinic telling me that no matter what the results were, we could handle this.

There was no beating around the bush.

The breast surgeon told us that unfortunately the biopsy taken from my right breast had come back with a positive diagnosis for cancer. It was estrogen and progesterone positive, which meant that the estrogen and progesterone in my body were feeding the growth of the tumour. Damn, I got it just for being a woman!

The invasive, ductal, stage two, grade one carcinoma (tumour tissue) had been hibernating in my right breast.

Invasive: *meaning the cancer cells have invaded or spread to the surrounding tissue*
Ductal: *in the milk duct*
Stage 2: *there are four stages*
Grade one: *the speed at which cancer grows; there are only three grades, one being the slowest*
Carcinoma: *cancer*

It was sitting in one of my milk ducts and, just to add insult to injury, it had leaked out and partnered up with a lymph node in my right armpit.

Boom! Cancer. My body had let me down. Or had I let it down? I sat confused. I knew that we all have cancer cells inside of us (oncogenes), but I also knew that they had to be triggered to grow. Did I trigger it? If I did, what was that trigger? I couldn't be sure, but what I was sure of was that I would do everything in my power to eradicate this cancer. I didn't invite it in; it just barged right in! I was neither angry nor scared, but I know I was quiet and instantly numb.

I was appalled to find out that 'it' had got me. It wasn't supposed to get me. Not me. I was catapulted into the medical world so quickly it made my head spin. I always saw the glass half full – always. But it wasn't until the *Big C* came along that I realised this attitude was about to be challenged.

Life's rose-coloured glasses had splintered. Hearing the diagnosis was the start of my thinking that life just might not be the bed of roses I thought it was. Cancer was about to change the course of my life.

With our family history, I should've known what some of the 'doctor speak' meant, but that would be a stretch of the truth. I knew that stage zero and stage one meant that a mass would be small and only found in one spot (*in situ*); stage two would be a bit bigger; stage three meant it would be reasonably larger and might've started to spread into surrounding tissue; and stage four meant it had spread from the original site and out of the lymph nodes, potentially being found in the bones, the liver, the lungs or the brain.

I admit I didn't hear most of what the breast surgeon said to me. I was busy managing the 'white noise'. When I eventually became present in the conversation again, I heard her ask, 'So, do you have any questions?' I replied, 'No.' NO? What did I mean 'NO'? I've just had a cancer diagnosis and I said 'NO'. In my regular life, I ask questions all the time – I'm so curious.

Now for anyone who knows me, the fact that I said no will make them laugh. John looked at me in a special way which reminded me that I had formed a few questions in case the appointment didn't go the way we'd hoped. Thank goodness for John! He absorbed the rest of what was said and filled me in later.

I'd become a member of a club to which I didn't want to belong. What I have learned, is that the first rule of cancer club is: don't *ever* worry about asking too many questions.

One thing that I was *very, very* sure of that day was that at some point I *needed* my breasts surgically removed. The twins had to go. In my head, electing to remove my breasts would give me the best chance of living a longer life. It was a very personal but very easy decision to make.

I had been with John at this point for twenty-five years and my breasts had fed both of my babies. Their work was done. During the first meeting, I confidently requested a prophylactic bilateral mastectomy.

> **prophylactic:** *intended to prevent disease*
> **bilateral:** *affecting both sides*
> **mastectomy:** *surgical operation to remove breast tissue*

I knew this was something I would have to wait for and my breast surgeon knew, with her experience, that I would still need a lumpectomy fairly urgently – a surgical removal of the tumour and some surrounding tissue. This would be followed up with some precautionary radiation therapy. She'd also set up a meeting for me with a Peninsula-based medical oncologist to discuss the possibility of shutting down my ovaries using a medication called tamoxifen, with the eventual removal of my ovaries.

She finished the consultation by letting me know that the cancer was small, they had caught it early, and she'd like me to see a cosmetic surgeon in the city to discuss the future mastectomy I'd requested. I remember thinking, *Wow, that is a lot of people for something so small.*

My breast surgeon was looking at the bigger picture and I was grateful. I knew that when I saw her next, I would have so many more questions. My next move was sorting out my private health insurance to manage this situation. I am a true believer in having health insurance and had held various policies for over eighteen years.

Once outside, John stopped and gave me the biggest, warmest hug I'd had for a while and we held hands tightly. In that moment, moulded in that embrace, life seemed so fragile. On the drive home I could feel the nervous tension. John's humour took a back seat and mine totally switched off. Life had just changed direction. Humour was the constant in our relationship, always had been, but not today. We were both deep in thought. What the hell had just happened?

Before we entered our home, he held me close, reassuring me that even though it was cancer, it was an invasive ductal carcinoma, a very common cancer, and with that came experience. The doctors would know *exactly* how to get rid of it.

I noticed our friends Mandy and Rich's car outside our home. Inside, they were there sharing a cuppa and a chat with Ginny, who was propped up at the kitchen bench with her laptop while our children were quietly watching TV in the lounge room. Ginny silently signalled to me – thumbs up or thumbs down? I responded silently with the appropriate sign. She turned her head away with pursed lips.

I immediately went to the fridge to get the bottle of expensive champagne that I'd won at my children's recent school trivia night. I wasn't a regular drinker, but today it was bubbles for dinner. As I moved around the kitchen looking for champagne flutes, John took Mandy and Rich out onto the back decking to tell them where we'd been. They were horrified.

MANDY:

'A few days before the diagnosis, Lindsey and I got together to do what we do best – drink tea excessively and eat lunch. It's the English in us – tea, tea and more tea. We sat down on the couch and she

seriously looked at me and said she needed to talk. Lindsey told me they had found a lump in her breast and then the other words that every woman never wants to hear about her closest friend, "It might be breast cancer." My world stopped. She was talking to me, but all I could do was watch her beautiful face trying to be brave. I knew she was doing this to be strong for me. Only Lindsey would be thinking of someone else at this time.

My next thought was, "If it is cancer, we will fight this together." It was then she told me that the lump had been discovered on 25th January. I couldn't believe she knew the day she had celebrated with me becoming an Australian citizen, that she'd sat there laughing and chatting, not sharing her news because she didn't want to spoil my celebration day. What a woman!

Not long after, John told us the results as Lindsey got the cham-pagne glasses out, as she wanted bubbles! The words stuck in John's throat as he confirmed to us that it was, in fact, breast cancer. Rich's grip tightened. I immediately wanted to hug her and tell her it would be okay, but I couldn't as their children didn't know yet.

Lindsey's cancer journey had begun. Behind her was a huge team of family and friends ready to go into battle with her, ready to support her, John and the kids. I got that hug eventually from my friend, my Aussie sister, whom I love dearly. And I was right – everything turned out all right, a little bit bumpier than expected, but all right.'

We needed time to absorb this new information so we decided not to tell the children until we had a solid plan. When our friends had left, I knew I had a very difficult task to complete and this one would prove the hardest of the lot. I had to tell my family, in particular, my parents and Roisin.

I video-called them and, in the most jovial manner, the words flowed from my mouth. I joked about how they were going to be cancer experts by the end of this and told them that I was sorry they had to go through all this… again. Mum was teary and Dad was stoic, but I could see the pain behind his eyes. I then set a mission for them – they had to get my sister over to their place so I could deliver the crappy news to her. We made a secret plan that Dad would *need* some potatoes from the supermarket in an attempt to steer her to their house.

Roisin and I are eight years and a little over 17,000 kilometres apart but we're always very well connected by our hearts. Let's face it – it was us two against four burly brothers. We always had to have each other's backs. I needed to tell her my news face to face and had to wait until the time difference would allow this. Pacing my decking for the longest time, I felt like a restless tiger in the zoo in anticipation of what was ahead of me. Breathing deeply and with John by my side, and Mum and Dad in on the plan, I dialled.

Roisin appeared on the screen, full face of make-up, glowing and happy. God, this was going to be hard. A passenger in the car, she was singing along to the radio and over-gesticulating with her head and hands. *I can't ruin her day*, I thought. *I just can't.* Luckily, she told me that she was about to pull up outside the supermarket and that they were going to be home in an hour. It was ten o'clock at night in Australia and I knew we were getting up early to drive to the airport. I left it for an hour and the plan worked. She arrived at my parents, saw me on the call, and settled in for a chinwag.

Looking down the lens, feeling a million miles away from anyone, I spent the next few minutes outlining to Roisin what had happened from beginning to end. All the while I could see the furrowed brows of Mum, Dad and Michael Brown staring down the phone. In that call, I thanked my sister. I thanked her for her second diagnosis. Without that I would've left my breast check for much longer because 'I was very busy, you know' and I'd already got the all-clear not that long ago. She had pressed and I had listened.

She was angry at our news. No, furious. Was this a joke? A bad dream? As if it could happen again to us! What the hell was going on? I remained positive and told her how lucky I was that I had her experience, unfortunately, to draw on. The heavy conversation turned light after she asked, 'So, you didn't really need potatoes, Dad?'

I ended the call heartbroken, only just holding myself together. The pendulum swung again later that day and I found myself imagining our children's lives without a mum. It was torture. I was terrified, but as usual John stepped up and grounded me. It was so unfortunate that Roisin and I were diagnosed with cancer at the same time, but he was strangely grateful and secure in the fact that she had potentially helped to save my life. John and I talked until very late in the night and finally fell asleep holding hands.

ROISIN:

'I had a video-call from Lindsey, but I was busy, as usual. She said she'd just call back later. I thought nothing of it. I thought she was just calling to talk about her trip over – she had booked a ticket the minute she'd heard about my recurrence.

I'd contacted her earlier in the month to tell her my bastard cancer was back. I hated having to tell her when we were so far apart. The first time I was diagnosed with breast cancer in 2014, I'd done the same – called to tell her the shitty news. She responded like I knew she would…"This is dreadful, but let's do this. I'm coming home." When I told her about my recurrence, I expected something similar. But this time, I said to her, "Oh Lins, I'm so sorry. I've got some rubbish news." Her eyes panicked and I could see the alarm bells ringing. I just blurted it out and told her my breast cancer was back. She just burst into tears… sobbed while miles and miles away from me in a place where I couldn't reach out to her, hug her or hold her hand. It was horrific.

I had arrived at my parent's place and they were keen to make me stay for a cuppa. They told me Lindsey was on video-call. They'd planned for me to be there so they could look after me when I heard the news. "Eya luvvvvvvv," we chimed!

To me, she looked happy as she sat with John. She told me she had some news and I, 1,000% did not expect what she was about to tell me. She went on to say she'd been for a mammogram and I started to wonder where she was going with this. Then she told me the bad news and my stomach dropped to the floor, and I literally felt my heart break. I knew there's no way she would play a joke like this on me, but somehow it just seemed impossible. My poor Lindsey, all that way away. I was devastated.

I knew the fear she would've been going through in the days before she told us and the fear now, knowing what was to come. I knew how her heart would've been hurting every time she looked at her children, and I especially knew how difficult that video-call to me would've been.

Our poor parents. I couldn't bear that they were going through this with their third child. How much could they take? It just didn't seem fair. We were so frustrated this absolute nightmare was unfolding.

My whole life, Lindsey had been a wonderful big sister. She mothered me whether I liked it or not, and now I felt such a strong urge to protect her. I had been through this once already, I was a pro at cancer now, so I took small comfort being able to fully understand the fears, the sickness and the devastation she felt.

Once Lindsey had gotten over the initial shock, she pulled her fighting pants right up to wedgie level and started kicking ass! I was so proud of her. My hero! We understood when we didn't hear from each other for a couple of days because we were too unwell with the awful side effects, and we celebrated each other coming out of our dark days.'

The next day, John left to fly to Queensland for three weeks. No matter what the breast surgeon had revealed, he had to go. We trusted that the specialists were busy putting together a solid plan and, even with John being away, I knew that I had enough of a social network to manage those delicate three weeks. We told our children that their school principal had allowed me to work from home while John was away – an essential white lie that bought us the time we needed.

Before dawn, we set off for Tullamarine Airport with two sleepy children in the car. Holding hands the whole way there, we didn't talk much. We promised each other to be in touch every day and that we'd tell the children when we were ready. After quick goodbyes to avoid a meltdown, I drove back to Frankston feeling really nauseous. Previously, John and I had been apart before for several weeks, but this was different. I now had three weeks on my hands with only the children to look after and appointments to go to, and the task of letting my Australian family and friends know.

One thing that I knew would be dangerous for me was researching online. When my sister was diagnosed, she took to using the internet to learn all about cancer, but I simply didn't feel like it. There was too much to know, too much about cancer for me to even think about researching. It was a complex topic and I felt completely overwhelmed by it all. Everything was there for me at the click of a button. I could access anything I wanted, but I was too angry to give it my attention. I was happier to place my trust in the many specialists who were about to consume my world.

I had to leave my car at the local repair shop due to a minor car accident and I was given a brand new red Kia to zip around in. It was met with squeals of delight when I tricked the children that I'd won it in a competition, then I was promptly scolded after confessing the truth! I had a huge belly laugh and, catching my reflection in the mirror, I loved the short-lived feeling. We drove around visiting as many people as we could, primarily to get out and about, but also to keep my mind occupied.

Not long after, I went to see a local psychic. To this day, I don't know why I did it, but I had been to one before about nine years ago (at the time of writing this) and loved it. I guess I was searching for some kind of understanding of my current situation. I settled into her huge comfortable couch, eager for information. I was amazed how much she knew about me! She was on the money for the most part, but the hour passed with no mention of illness or sickness, which, if I'm honest, was the sole reason I went in the first place.

I drove home wondering why cancer had not been sensed or been at the core of the reading, then it hit me! Psychics are not supposed to tell you bad things. Oh no, was I going to die? Then something else dawned on me. I remembered she'd asked my name at the time of the booking. What if she had just looked at my online social media? That was it! She had checked my socials! No wonder she was on the money. More like all about the money, a true fake, and I felt conned and completely taken advantage of. Never again, no more psychics. I just had to deal with whatever life served me.

My breast surgeon had organised a pelvic ultrasound. I assumed it was because breast cancer and gynaecological cancers can be linked. I had never had one before and was expecting just a bit of ultrasound gel on my stomach and a little check of my ovaries. WRONG! It was nothing short of a large wand covered in a plastic bag inserted into my personal area. I wanted it to be over so much! Thankfully, the results came back clear.

I remember driving home and every time I saw a female, I would hope that she had been for a check-up. It's strange to admit, but I started staring at many breasts and worrying about them. I wondered how many women were walking around with scarred boobs, implants, expanders or no boobs. I felt like I should be wearing a t-shirt reading, 'Have you checked your boobs?' An irrational thought maybe? Maybe not? I didn't realise it at the time, but now upon reflection, I was experiencing very high levels of stress. My arms, at times, still didn't work properly and I was simply not myself.

Word had slowly spread in my circle of family and friends that I was unwell, which was strange because, in the mirror I looked totally fine. B.J., one of my neighbours and a school dad, was unfortunately diagnosed with cancer the year before I was, but had done a royal job at beating this dreadful disease. He visited not long after he heard my bad news and offered me not only sound advice, but booklets from the Cancer Council (www.cancer.org. au) filled with how to delicately tell children about a diagnosis. Poor guy! I reckon I chewed his ear off for three hours. He became the one to answer my barrage of early questions that I hadn't asked anyone else yet. I was grateful that he'd taken the time out to be with me that day. He was great and I loved the feeling of community that was to soon wrap its arms delicately around me.

One of first things I needed when diagnosed was to reach out to learn from other women who had survived breast cancer. Hearing positive stories were so vital for my mental state at this time. I needed experiences to which I could deeply relate, so I reached out to Cindy's mum, Sylvie. This was an attempt to hear how you can live through breast cancer and still manage to 'glow' afterwards.

The way she spoke about her cancer was so uplifting. She took a laid-back approach with it and the tone of her voice left me feeling comforted. Looking back, I felt it prepared me for the road ahead and I remain eternally grateful to her. I left the house feeling positive, as Sylvie's overall message was clear: yes, cancer had happened, it was worrying for a time, not to mention stressful, but just stay positive and believe that things will be okay in the end. I was assured that you can endure health issues – even something as scary as cancer – but that you can also go on to live a happy, healthy life too. I grabbed this idea and ran with it.

Over the three weeks without John, I would catch glimpses of Layla's and Lennox's faces and burst out crying. I cried secretly in the shower because it was out of everybody's way. If they asked, a white lie would naturally happen: 'I got shampoo in my eyes' or 'I bumped myself getting out of the shower.' It worked every time.

From the moment Layla was born I have adored her. She is kind to everyone, hilarious and a mini social justice warrior. She also has the conversation skills of an adult and a smile that is difficult not to reciprocate. John and I are often complimented on the fact that she's so brilliant. Lennox is equally kind to all he comes across and has the energy levels to put The Roadrunner to shame. His sharp wit runs rings around many and he makes me double over in laughter most days.

At this stage, I took the time to have some 'me time'. I drove to Dromana, a place that we love to visit as a family. For me, Dromana holds lovely memories of family time, joy, beach and delicious ice-cream. Looking out to sea, I contemplated how I was going to get through this, not in a, 'How am I ever going to get through this' sense – more of a 'What do I have to do to fight this thing' way, and it was there on the bench that my metaphorical boxing gloves went on. I told myself there was always someone worse off and not for one second was I prepared to think about the 'd' word – death. In my head, I replayed affirmations over and over that I'd read on social media and which I knew would help me.

'It's not what we have in life, but who we have in life that matters.' J.M. Laurence

'Wake up every morning and tell yourself you can do this.' Zig Ziglar

'When you are in a dark place, you sometimes tend to think you have been buried. Perhaps you have been planted. Bloom.' Christine Caine

For the finale on the bench that day, I finished with, 'Cancer, you picked the wrong lady!'

When I met with my breast surgeon again, it had been a little over a week since the news of the lump in my breast. Inquiring as to how long the lump had been there playing the nasty game of multiplication inside me, the answer was, 'No one knows. That's the one thing I can't answer.' This was hard to take and equally frustrating because I had been asymptomatic. Leaving her consulting rooms, I wondered if she thought about me as a person – my identity, my values – or was it all about the job at hand?

Fairly quickly, I met with my appointed plastic surgeon in his office on Collins Street in Melbourne's central business district to discuss a long-term plan for me. I was again supported by my beautiful friend, Mandy, as John was still away. She drove, made me laugh all the way there, and it was a relaxed atmosphere that morning. The surgeon displayed a sensitive manner and walked me through all my options. His competent approach made me feel instantly happy with him and he thought it would be in my best interests to reduce my breast size (non-cancerous side) following my lumpectomy and in preparation for my mastectomy. There was the possibility post-lumpectomy that my breasts would be different sizes and it meant they'd be in a better shape post-mastectomy. I agreed. I had always been large chested and was pleased with the fact that I would eventually be smaller.

He also decided there and then that breast implants would not be an option. This was because with my brother, Sean, having suffered a form of lymphoma (cancer of the immune system), I'd be at risk of developing Breast Implant Associated Lymphoma – a type of non-Hodgkin lymphoma. Considering my family history, the surgeon just didn't want to take that risk.

He went on to talk me through a procedure called a D.I.E.P. with immediate reconstruction. It was a lot to take in and I was glad Mandy was there to pick up what I didn't. This surgery was going to be *huge*. D.I.E.P. stood for Deep Inferior Epigastric Procedure. Methodically yet simply, he outlined what it was, giving me information about timeframes, recovery and what the final result might look like. Put simply, he was going to take some tissue from my abdomen while my breast surgeon performed a double mastectomy, then he would replant the tissue onto my chest, transferring fat to form two new, warm, functional breasts made entirely of me.

Time was on my side. I had to now focus on the job at hand-kicking cancer into the middle of next week. I left fairly happy, but the surgery seemed a million miles away. I should have left it there, but instead, I did the unthinkable. I looked at D.I.E.P. online. I Dr. Googled! Nope, nah, not ever should I have done that. I should've gone with the 'ignorance is bliss' attitude and simply not looked.

My medical team worked in conjunction with each other. I knew multi-disciplinary meetings were held because of Roisin's past experiences, and I realised that was to happen to me. I saw them as allying with each other to help me not only get rid of my cancer, but to do all they could to make sure it did not come back again!

Feeling optimistic, I booked in with the secretary to jump the first hurdle and have the lumpectomy done a week later. Not too long before I would have NO cancer in my body. Wait! How would I know that? Will I get scans, CT's, bloodwork? How will I be certain it has all gone? Who was going to tell me I didn't have cancer anymore?

A few hours later, I received a phone call from the cosmetic surgeon's secretary with surprising and stressful news. Apparently, I wasn't covered by my insurance for the surgeries. WHAT? I remained composed on the phone, but inside my adrenalin was peaking. I was so disheartened. I wanted to scream. I didn't have the whizz-bang bells and whistles top cover that my health insurer could offer. It turns out this was the only way I could've had my mastectomy. What a blow! It felt like a second diagnosis.

I asked her for a rough figure as to how much it would cost me if I just used my savings and paid for it as I felt I needed to get that cancer out of my body and soon. I could feel the sting in my eyes as my mind flashed back to the photos of my children in my study. I *had* to be cancer-free. The secretary was amazing and probably didn't realise that the next conversation she was about to have with me would dramatically shape my life moving forward.

She told me that it would be fine to pay cash and go ahead with the surgery privately, but if anything were to go wrong, for example, if I ended up in intensive care or needed long-term care, I would probably come off worse. She informed me that people lose their homes in extreme cases, while others acquire insurmountable debt. She was never to know the impact of that conversation.

Decision made, I was to hop over to the public health system and be placed on a waiting list. Wow! I had paid health insurance for years in Australia and was devastated to think that now, the one time I needed it, I didn't have it. I never played sport so I'd never succumbed to injury, didn't tap into my policy extras, had minimal dental work, and had only had one surgery in my forty-four years of life. My friend, Kerryn, a health professional herself, popped in for a cuppa and was a real 'ear' for me later that day. She reassured me that this nightmare would be over soon and that I wouldn't be on the waiting list for long, not with cancer. I loved her timing and my manic panic was quickly over. It would take a further twenty-four *long* days for me to have that lumpectomy.

During this time, I invested in a plain white box to keep the mounting cancer documents in, which I hid in the wardrobe. I didn't want our children to stumble upon anything that could raise suspicion or cause unnecessary worry. When my family would call or text, I transformed into a stealthy burglar retreating onto my decking to chat so as not to be heard. I was alert and constantly on guard. I wanted to craft the right conversation before telling our children my dirty little secret. I knew it would have to be sooner rather than later.

I chose to tell my close friends over the phone. Calling was the best way for me because I couldn't bear to see the hopelessness in their eyes because I knew the pain of someone looking into my eyes and telling me they had cancer all too well.

It's worth mentioning here that charities helped me and my family ride the wave of cancer directly after diagnosis and beyond. Charities are a great resource you can trust because they deal with facts – not guessing or unsubstantiated information that can sometimes come with forums or social media.

I tapped into Breast Cancer Network Australia – BCNA – because I just wanted facts; they would aid me in making future decisions. Its role is to support both men and women all over Australia in what can be their darkest hours. They don't do research of any kind; rather, they support us by informing us, connecting us and representing us. They are change-makers, and they ask for better treatment and care to improve the journey for us. They also give us power with fact-based knowledge and information so we can always be our own best advocate. Additionally, they let us know the statistics in and around the topics of incidence, survival, mortality and risk. Knowledge is power, and I latched on to their website to find inner peace and strength. My wellbeing was certainly nurtured by reading positive accounts on BCNA, along with music, energy from friends, my support group, family and social media.

I also tapped into other wonderful charities such as Camp Quality www.campquality.org.au Think Pink www.thinkpink.org.au and Mummy's Wish www.mummyswish.org.au. I couldn't recommend highly enough reaching out in these early days. Sure, there were times I wanted to cry my bloody heart out and smack my hands on the wall like a madwoman, but I kept it under wraps with reason and deep breathing. I hid it inside and hoped that it wouldn't manifest into something bigger at a later date. I'm pleased to say it didn't. I attribute some of this to the professionalism of the charities and organisations set up to help people like me take on the battle that is cancer.

So, how do I cope with the emotional side of things? I talk. Plain and simple. Talking it out allows me to process what is happening. John is my best listener and he's the only one to whom I have disclosed my worst fears. Even then there are thoughts and feelings that not even he knows, because frankly, they are too scary to verbalise.

I also have sticky-note funerals. A sticky-note funeral is for whenever I have a scary thought, a frightening thought or a thought that threatens my wellbeing. I write it down on a yellow post-it note, read it aloud and then I rip it up into tiny pieces before throwing it in the bin. It works for me and is oh-so satisfying!

Four

The longest wait

*'Even now, as broken as you may feel, you are still so strong.
There's something to be said for how you hold yourself
together and keep moving, even though you feel like
shattering. Don't stop. This is your healing. It doesn't have
to be pretty or graceful. You just have to keep going.'*
Maxwell Diawuoh

No symptoms, no warning, just a screeching halt. A right turn, a forever change.

Stage 2?? That's half-way to dead. The pendulum swings.

After diagnosis, I would ask myself, *Am I in for a future of uncertainty now?* I would regret the thought almost immediately, telling myself I was stronger than that. As the days went by, I'd think, *Oh, a back niggle. Has the cancer spread in my spine now?* Then, as quickly as I had thought it, I'd alter my mindset and think, *Drop the drama, don't be silly. It's just a sore back.*

I have lost count as to how many flips I've done, convinced that I've had an undiagnosed toe, thumb, back, ear, liver and kidney cancer three times over. It takes a lot of mental strength to talk yourself out of that! I was the one who was never going to get sick, remember? However, I didn't want to live with the feeling of uncertainty. The unknown answers were toying with me. I *had* to change my inner dialogue.

Recently, I showed my children a short video of a male with a serious disability completing a gruelling forty-two-kilometre assault course. We watched in awe and reflected on how strong his mindset would have to be, not only to complete the course, but to *believe* he could complete it. Layla responded, 'You would have to have a solid mindset, Mum.' I felt fantastic hearing that. The tools that I used to build *me* were beginning to rub off on them. Being positive can be difficult, especially during times where emotions are conflicted or troublesome, but it's essential.

As the abundance of flowers and a steady flow of friends offering love, food parcels and small gifts arrived, we decided the time was right to tell our children. I had wondered if they'd sensed something was wrong – they certainly knew that things were different. Layla's social intelligence was high but at times, her anxiety was too, so I knew I had to tread carefully.

I used all my wellbeing skills and past teaching experiences of how to talk to children to orchestrate the conversation. John and I decided that the best-case scenario for us was to have John on video-call and for me to do the talking. Martine – a good friend I'd made because we'd lived on the same street for a year and formed a strong bond – had been over nearly every day at this point. She'd dropped in a little chocolate treat for both Layla and Lennox as she knew that I was going to tell them later that day. I called upon family to see who was available as I thought being surrounded by them after the fact would be a great distraction for the kids. I organised pizza and fun with the cousins. Nervous, I called John to see if he was free.

Cancer, unfortunately, was something with which Layla and Lennox were all too familiar. I began by telling them that Mummy had been to the doctor to have a breast check because of Aunty Roisin. I said that the doctor had found a very small lump in my breast (even if it was enormous, I still would've said the same) which had to come out, and that soon I would have a quick surgery… adding that I needed a doctor and a nurse to help make me better. I asked if they were up for the job. I kept it that brief.

There was a look of horror on Layla's face and she asked, 'Mum, do you have cancer?' There was no fooling her. I wasn't about to lie, sugar-coat it or be dramatic. The word bounced around the inside of my mouth resting on my tongue. I replied, 'Yes' and then quickly tried to cuddle her, but she pulled away, curled up into the foetal position and just sobbed. In fact, she howled, 'WHY? WHY? WHY YOU? WHY MY MUM? THAT IS THE

LAST THING I EXPECTED YOU TO SAY. THIS IS THE WORST DAY OF MY LIFE!'

Choking on tears, she hit me with the big one, 'MUUUUM, ARE YOU GOING TO DIE?'

Now, here's the thing. Ever since Layla uncovered the truth about childhood 'beliefs', we had a pact never to lie to each other. I found my mind wandering and my hand rubbing her back. I had to think, and quick.

The truth was, I didn't know the answer. I could die, I suppose – people do. So, what do I say? I hadn't expected such a strong reaction or rehearsed what I might say if she asked. I found it came very naturally to me to think incredibly positively, so I told her that I would be in the hands of Melbourne's top doctors and nurses and I knew in my heart that it would all work out. I wanted to scream, 'Of course I'm not going to die from this. It won't kill me', but I couldn't at that moment. I explained it to them as a 'temporary detour' and that it was caught early which was the best possible news.

In my peripheral vision, I could see Lennox's eyes darting between myself and the chocolate. I also realised John was silently crying, but for me, things were going in slow motion. I asked Lennox if he was okay and he responded with something that made me laugh out loud. 'Yeah Mum, I don't think you are going to die. Can I have the chocolate now, please?' He had his facts and now wanted to tap out of the conversation!! I motioned for him to go and play in the back garden with the family and prompted John to go back to work as I did not want Layla to see her dad crying. That would've tipped her over the edge.

I comforted Layla who, by this time, had calmed down somewhat. I think she'd just got a huge shock. I remember feeling angry – angry that she was too young to be coping with the news that I could no longer hide from them. I reassured her once again and out we went to be surrounded by family and lots and lots of cuddles. Putting the children to bed that night was hard and my throat burned trying to stifle my tears. Meditation music purred in both bedrooms and kissing them goodnight was so very special. I examined every inch of their young faces and held their small hands as they slept.

There it was, glaringly obvious and the major reason to fight.

JOHN:

'The video-call back to Melbourne when I was away in Queensland when we had to tell the children was probably the hardest thing I have ever had to do. Later that night I was consoled by the fact that the cancer was treatable and beatable. I still felt scared though. I haven't given any thought about it having the capacity to be fatal. I just won't allow any of those thoughts in. I've tried to stay very 'matter of fact' in the way it has to be treated and that whatever option Lindsey was going to choose for her body, I was going to support her, no matter what.'

Michael, another brother (I have a few), was always seen as the sacred brother. Mum even made the front page of the local newspaper holding her bundle of joy as he was the first baby born on Christmas Day that year. I recall how utterly beautiful my mum looked in the picture. She was radiant and certainly not what my mirror reflected after I'd given birth!

Michael is the most loyal, kind-hearted human you could ever meet – constantly a source of trust and always the one who would give you his last dollar. I was nine when he was born and I still have a special spot for our Christmas baby. He has three children of his own and is highly independent, happily working as a support assistant to troubled teens. Despite the miles between us, conversation with him always lifts my mood. We talked through how to manage what our children were facing and I particularly loved one of his suggestions – that I place diaries, pens and jars by Layla and Lennox's beds in case they wanted to offload any heavy burdens. I took to printing off positive affirmations for them. I think this helped them forge resilience and I saw it as helping them deal with it.

Roisin had said that she was going to kick cancer's ass as she was in the 'strong girls' club'. Layla asked if I was in it. I told her I was the president of it and invited her to join. She looked at me and said, 'But I haven't got cancer.' That night the strong girls' club got bigger. We messaged my mum and Roisin's daughter, Ivy (now aged four), and there it was. The strong girls club now had five new members and a new club rule: you didn't have to have cancer to get in!

With all my family on board looking out for us, here I was thinking that telling our children had gone really well. A couple of months later, Layla came out of her room waving a magazine that a charity had mailed me, shouting, 'Now I get it, Mum' which was strange, as I thought she already had got it. It was her little lightbulb moment. Fabulous – I didn't want the children not to be informed. Being scared and worried under such circumstances was normal, but I also wanted them to be on board the 'positive mindset train'.

I knew surgery could be any day and I sat by the phone, waiting. It turned out to be the longest wait where I swayed wildly between thinking *Australia is one of the best countries to get sick, I'll be fine*, to *Why did I get it?* It was as if I was trying to solve a puzzle – one I knew in the back of my mind I would never solve. As part of this, I would review my life choices many times over, often when I was alone, and I'd do it on a very deep level. I knew I was a 'category one urgent' on the waiting list, but I remained a public patient and a wait was inevitable. It was weird. I felt well, but at the same time, I knew this was a super serious situation.

I waited and waited and waited. I called admissions almost daily to find out if I had a surgery date, aware that I was being a pest, but not too worried about that because I had a family for whom I needed to be around. Panic began to build and my U.K. family members were starting to feel uneasy. After days of waiting, I finally had my first surgery date. It was to be in five days. February 27th. I needed new slippers and underwear. I had to present well for surgery after all. Mum always taught me to wear clean undies, in case you were in a car accident. No one wants the doctors to have a bad shift!

I recall sitting in a café with Cindy happily chatting about how everything would go back to normal after the lumpectomy, until I have the mastectomy and, even then, it would be a six-week recovery. I never wanted to be that cancer patient who cried in despair or got depressed, and I worked very hard not to be that person. Being positive was like medicine for my soul – it helped me on the dark days and it made me feel hopeful.

I had decided I was going to let my principal know that she should perhaps replace my contact hours in the classroom. It would be unfair to the school as I couldn't offer consistency at this time. I'd been working in leadership for the last few years but remained the art teacher in a part-time role. It was decided that I would be ideal to work as a casual relief teacher for that year, in and around my two surgeries. That doesn't mean I was comfortable with the idea of someone else having my job. I loved it, especially the contact time with the children – they were the whole reason why I became a teacher in the first place. But it was something that had to be done. It was to be the end of my full-time teaching career but I knew I would be back casually sometime soon.

I started to feel unwell over the next few days and, disappointingly, I had to give away some Missy Higgins concert tickets. I was already worried about future missed opportunities, so I stopped booking any activities as I simply didn't know where I would be in my recovery. Life became alarmingly unpredictable. Roisin suggested writing down two things I wanted to do when I was better for every one event missed. I loved this idea and embraced it. I also worried about cash flow, but was left feeling reassured by John. I had to face it – I was unwell. I was gutted that illness had got in the way of my fun. Being a busy working mum of two meant that I didn't get out much. The concert signified the first of many cancellations to come.

My friend, Naomi, a wellbeing fountain of knowledge, popped in not long after this, reminding me that all this crap was temporary and that I'd be out and about soon enough. As more friends came to know what was going on in our family, people were coming over for hot tea and warm conversation. Tea became a theme in our house. I found myself investing in many different teas and I drank a lot of tea from this point on. I figured it was better than wine, right? There is something special about wrapping your hands around a hot mug of something. I am married to someone who doesn't drink anything hot, which I find strange, but on the upside, I only ever have to make one cup of tea. I knew I had a fabulous support network and I was certain there would be a lot of future kettle-boiling going on.

It's funny how the universe repays you. One day, in my 'old life' as I like to call it, I met a lady shading from the heat of an Australian summer's day under a tree at the school where I'd been working. I chatted with Mel and we immediately connected. She had just arrived from New Zealand and I found myself asking her questions just to hear her accent. She mentioned that she was in education and was looking for a job. I passed her resumé onto my principal and she employed her not long after. I was thrilled. We became good pals after that and I'm so grateful for her for many reasons. She has held my hand so many times over the last couple of years and I didn't quite realise that this was a friendship that would flourish with steely pace.

MEL:

'Friends come and go in life, ties slowly unthread or wear beyond repair. This is not one of those stories. Lindsey is my whirlwind friend. In a very short time we became close, and in that time she has taught me the true meaning of friendship. I love her energy, her compassion, the way she sees the positive in everyone and her laugh, OMG, her laugh!

I've never spoken the following out loud because, in my head, I feel it is very selfish and I don't want it to sound like this is all about me, but, for the purpose of this book, I think we need to acknowledge that the cancer tsunami reaches far beyond the impact zone. Some may be able to make a meal, say a prayer and then leave the mind-numbing anger at the front gate, returning to the ho-hum of day-to-day life. Not me.

I had never known cancer. The whole time, as I was developing a bond with this amazing woman, it was cruelly trying to steal my new friend away. When it finally presented its ugly face, I knew I had to prepare to fight for Lindsey…. How dare it try to take her from me!

I became proactive and did what I knew best. I cooked. I decided to be that practical friend. Each meal I made, I cried. My favourite and worst part of the meals was dropping them off. I wanted to see Lindsey, be with her, laugh with her. I wanted my friend and felt I didn't know how to be a good friend to her now. I was too consumed by thoughts… those ones we lock away such as, 'What if?', 'When?' and 'How will?' Lindsey would be telling me about her 'Where to next?' and I wouldn't hear a thing. I mean, I was listening, but I was incapable of taking any of it in. Cancer was winning. It was screwing with my mind.

I decided to put more energy into the kids. I helped out where I could with pick-up and drop-off. I took the beautiful Layla and Lennox out, had them over for playdates and sleepovers, even taught Layla to cook the family favourite meal! I was trying to distract myself as much as I was them. 'Can I call Mum, just to check in?' I will never forget their little faces in these moments. I could see pain in their eyes. I know I am a little bit braver and a little bit wiser because I have Lindsey in my life. I am so grateful that this friendship is to be continued...'

It was about this time I started to think about what I could do or what I needed to do in order to NEVER get cancer again, so I called Roisin for some tips. She had been newly diagnosed as stage 3C, which was a horrible shock as her previous cancer had only been stage 2 (and although I didn't know it at the time, she'd been told the cancer was advanced and could only be managed and not cured).

I knew I had to change some of my health habits, but not too much as I thought I was doing quite well at looking after myself and my family. I reached a point where I thought that's it: no sugar, no alcohol and more greens, but immediately thought, *I love chocolate,* and in the height of summer, I loved the feeling of having a cold beer on the back deck with John. I had to find a happy medium.

After a conversation with my sister outlining what she was doing, I opened up my pantry and filled a large bin liner with stuff I knew probably shouldn't be there and, if I'm being honest with myself I knew that, for the most part, it was there for 'convenience'. As a busy working mum, it had been easier to pop something in the oven. I donated the removed food to the homeless and decided to dramatically reduce sugary treats.

On the drive home from school pick-up that day, Lennox asked, 'Do I still have to do no sugar when you finish with this cancer?' Day one and he was already checking! I explained that it was called a lifestyle change and that we would all become a little bit more mindful of how we were treating our bodies. It was at dinner that night that Layla asked if cancer was contagious. Wow! I was so proud of both our children. They were being so open and allowing me and John in to view some of their emotional baggage. We were in this together.

I was starting to learn of the profound effect cancer can have on those close to us. That weekend, we made a roast dinner with Brussel sprouts on the menu. I don't like Brussel sprouts, but I knew that they were really good for you, high in nutrients and rich in antioxidants, so I roasted them in olive oil and garlic. Lennox declared with a perfectly formed face of disgust, 'It's not fair, I haven't got cancer. I shouldn't have to eat all these Brussel sprouts.' It made us all roll with laughter, something that we did often at the dinner table. I explained to him that our focus now had to be on wellness, not illness, and that delicious foods would act as our medicine. Change was in order in our home. We were to remove preservatives and add more things that grew on trees or in the ground. It was a lot for eight and ten year-olds to take in.

Over the next few days, I started to do strange things. I used my negative energy to spring clean the house from top to bottom. I realised I was mimicking a typical 'nesting' behaviour, not too dissimilar to pregnant women. I wasn't working so I had time to tidy and sort, and deep down I knew I'd be out of action at home for a number of weeks so that was enough reasoning for me. This had to happen to get the house ready to make life as easy as possible for John.

I began to train Layla and Lennox to take on more responsibility in the house in an attempt to limit chaos. I shopped online for groceries, pre-paid my bills, had my car serviced and had a scale and clean at the dentist. I ran that house and I knew I had to hand the reins over, which was stressful because, at times, I could be a massive control freak. I just needed a sense of control in my life and a feeling of order as my world was about to be thrust upside down.

I received a phone call from my breast surgeon later that day asking me to come in and fill out some documentation for my operation. That bloody pendulum! The highs and lows were very unpredictable. On the short drive there, I started to think about raising more cancer awareness in my social circle. People were aware that breast cancer was the enemy and affected the lives of one in seven in Australia, but I wanted to get people checking themselves regularly, really regularly. I wanted to encourage free-flowing conversations where taboo subject matter was not even a thing. I wanted everyone to have open and honest conversations. I wanted to get people checking in on others.

Many of us spend more time with our work colleagues than our own immediate families. Colleagues can become like family. We always look out for family, right? Why did I want to do something? As John and I had made the joint decision for me to not be at work, I *had* to have a purpose, some kind of distraction, and to be honest, it just felt important to me. How I was going to do this I wasn't sure yet. I had to focus on me first.

Questions were coming thick and fast from visitors and our children, some of which I could answer, others I struggled with. 'Can you feel cancer?' 'Will you have to have chemotherapy?' 'What percentage of women that get it, die from it?' 'What's radiation therapy?' 'How does it work?' 'How do you know it's gone after your operation?' 'Will you get to see the tumour when they cut it out?' And the hardest one… 'Why did cancer choose you, Mum?'

Pass the tissues please.

One morning, Lennox crept into my room and gently woke me, asking if I wanted him to make me breakfast. He was such a caring little soul and I took him up on the offer of two pieces of Vegemite on toast. His parting message as he left to take part in 'operation breakfast' was, 'I just want to look after you, Mum.' Equally, Layla became very close to me physically and emotionally. She would often sit next to me on the sofa holding my hand. We were a tactile family by nature, but this was different. My phone would light up with messages of love and concern from my social circle and Layla made it her mission to read them out loud to me, reminding me of how beautiful and caring my family and friends were.

The stream of immediate support was endless. Mandy took me out for pedicures and shopping, Mel fed me, Martine came to appointments with me, and Cindy kept me laughing all the way through. I remember taking time to appreciate rosellas in the back garden and the beach at St Kilda – things I had seen many times before. Things just seem brighter. They sparkled. One of our close friends, 'Brassy', whom John had played soccer with for many years, took the time to drive down from his flower farm in Lilydale to deliver the largest bunch of flowers for both me and Layla – red for me and pink for Layla. I will never forget the size of that effort. He was truly devoted as a friend and both John and I looked upon the gesture highly. Here I was receiving all this attention, but I still felt just like me. There was no pain, no wounds and no blood; just a diagnosis. It was, once again, a strange paradox.

We took the time to carefully examine our paperwork. We had taken out life insurance about twelve years earlier, not for any particular reason other than the 'you never know' scenario. Thinking about composing a will led to feelings of despair, if I'm honest. John and I were each other's worlds and had been for a long time. I imagined life without me in it, and I don't mean that in a narcissistic kind of way… more in such a way that I planned out what life would be like without me in it. I imagined my funeral. I touched the small diamond necklace that I rarely took off, wondering if I would be buried in it. With a fine-tooth comb, I trudged through the rest of the day checking I had everything in order. I broke down more than once, but, by the end, I knew exactly what to write in our will, albeit a hard path to walk.

Our children came home from school one day and told me that they'd been sitting on the friendship bench at school. This brightly coloured bench is used predominantly for alerting teachers and other students that there might be a problem. It broke my heart that they were sad at school. My diagnosis was a lot for them to digest and I pondered over how much information to give them: *Have I been too honest? Have I told them too much? Do I involve them? Do I not?* I always knew I would have to let them know, but this forced me to think harder.

One thing I did know was to keep any information I gave them fact-based and let them come to me asking questions. I would be as honest as I could be and I was sure to drop any dramatics. Very early on, as soon as their school knew our situation, both children were offered a thirty-minute counselling session. I couldn't have been happier. What a great thing to have in place! I never asked Layla or Lennox about these sessions, but often they would come home and share what they said or did. I truly believed this made an obvious difference with how they managed my diagnosis and how well-balanced they seemed overall.

Lennox had begun begging to sleep in his sister's room, on the trundle bed. She definitely wasn't up for this and a battle ensued. Layla wasn't very needy at this point but evidently Lennox was. Now and again and under duress, she caved, leaving Lennox beaming from ear to ear. Layla remained angry at cancer and mostly needed downtime alone in her room. I was losing the lump and Layla was losing her faith. A cancer diagnosis had made Layla question God. Her poor little mind! She found it stressful wondering why these things 'just happen'. She wasn't alone.

Having been fairly mentally drained after the initial diagnosis, I soon found my mental state improving. It was getting stronger. I reasoned with myself by thinking that getting cancer was just a bit of bad luck and that it was just some time out from my regular life.

Shortly after this, I received some news that I knew would brighten all our days. My cousin, Roxy, was coming to Australia from England and bringing her five-month-old baby girl, Genie – a very welcoming and exciting distraction. She was nine years my junior, had been to Australia many times, even living with us for a year, and was a ball of fun. The nesting was about to pay off.

I picked Roxy and Genie up from Melbourne Airport with suitcases stuffed with gifts from my family and treats that we all missed from the U.K. Layla and Lennox did not want to go to school, due to Genie's cuteness overload. Roxy had left her two year-old at home with his dad to come over to see me, sit and laugh and reminisce, and I can never thank her enough. As we were going to school, Lennox called back over his shoulder, 'I hope *you* don't get cancer, Genie!' There he goes again!

Valentine's Day was on its way. John and I had only ever been apart on 'love day' once in our twenty-six years together. We always celebrated this special day and had definitely given in to the powers of commercialism to spoil each other. This time though, due to John being in Queensland, I passed the day by going to the movies, entertaining guests and spoiling myself by shopping for a new bed. It was a beautiful bed and somewhere that I would spend a fair bit of time over the next few years.

I consistently kept in touch with Roisin and Sean to seek advice and have a natter, but most of all, just to feel close to them. I was living so far away and it was tough. I thought about how my three undiagnosed brothers were feeling: Terry, the eldest, Tony, the tallest and Michael, the kindest. I wondered about when, on hearing of a fourth immediate family cancer diagnosis, if they thought of themselves as 'sitting ducks', but I was too scared to ask. I longed to be hugged. I mean, really hugged, a lengthy one, one where there is some back stroking or a bit of rocking and maybe some 'mmms' and 'ahhhs'. It made me smile and think of those funny free hugs videos from the internet.

At this time, I was on the path of discovery and made a very random decision: I would give acupuncture a go. It is used to stimulate energy imbalance and help pain, essentially placing it in the naughty corner until the reason for the pain is found. I had convinced myself that it would be invisible magic and would act as a muscle relaxant as my heavy arms continued to annoy me. Cindy raved about acupuncture and it didn't take long for me to track down a very reputable Chinese medicine doctor.

On my first appointment, I noticed he took what I thought was my pulse, but I realised that he was monitoring my blood flow. I watched his hands closely while he typed on the computer. He recorded 'consistent' for the left arm and much to my distress he typed 'choppy' for the right. Choppy? What did that mean?! It seemed to make sense, I suppose, that the cancer was on the right, but was it worse than I thought? Choppy. I still can't fathom that. He was a man of few words. After a brief history from me, he asked me to hop up on the bed. He then instructed me to tell him when I hit the point of pain while he placed what can only be described as small spears into sixteen different parts of my body. Sixteen! He then placed warm red lamps over my abdomen and my feet and left the room for around twenty-five minutes.

For a short time, I was Gulliver. I started to second guess why I was doing this, but reminded myself that I wasn't well at this point and I had to do whatever I could to help myself. Unexpectedly, tears fell and pooled in my ears but I didn't dare move for fear of one of those 'spears' going further in! I left with a bag of something that resembled forest floor findings, but held the promise of making me feel a bit better. On the way home, I continued to think about why I had gone there. I think I was trying to tap into natural therapies to feel like I was doing something.

The copious amount of appointments continued. John was due home from Queensland two days before my cancer removing surgery and my nerves were real, so I called on Roisin again for peace of mind. I knew it was perfectly okay for me to have these feelings. It feels like forever in the beginning. There are so many tests that need to be done and it's so time-consuming. The waiting is the hardest part and can be overwhelming. I would breathe deeply and write EVERYTHING down.

John returned and we sat down with my appointed medical oncologist the next day. She made both of us feel comfortable very quickly and discussed various elements and options for my future treatment. She initially mentioned genetic testing. I was in two minds about this. Sure, I had a daughter to think about but my sister had completed it and she came back negative for both the BRCA1 and the BRCA2 gene. We discussed the possibility of chemotherapy but that was highly unlikely as the tumour site appeared to be small. I chose to put it to the back of my mind.

I was on a very fast rollercoaster after hearing 'positive for cancer' and it was soon time to disembark. At times, it felt like I was in a dream from which I couldn't wake.

Five

Losing the lump

'There is no dignity with breast cancer. So many people
see so many parts of you on so many occasions!'
Rachelle Kregor

A tumour had grown and nested in an unwanted zone, pushing healthy tissue to the side to find room for its nasty wrongdoings. This tumour might be nasty, but I was ready to push back, hard. Finally, *the* pre-operative information phone call arrived. It was pre-op information along with an operation date. Excited, I called John. That day, I decided I would take some photographs of my chest and document the journey in pictures for as long as it took. On the journey home from any visit with a specialist of any kind, I would compile a list of questions on my phone for the next appointment to make sure I understood everything that was going to happen to me. This was my commitment to myself from the day of my diagnosis.

John and I attended the Nuclear Department of the hospital the day before my procedure to have a radioactive substance known as a tracer injected into my skin above and around the tumour, which, in my case was directly into the areola. This tracer is radioactive and spreads throughout the local lymphatic region. On the same day and into the same site, blue dye was also injected into the functional elements of the breast such as the lobules and ducts, and it rapidly spread. This dual method allows the surgeon to be highly accurate, and the tracer also marks where cancer cells may have left the breast and gone into the lymph nodes.

Arriving at the hospital, the nurse asked if I was okay and told me that the needle I was about to receive was a bit 'pinchy' and she hoped it went well. A second nurse also mentioned that the injection was 'full-on' and was probably going to hurt. Great! She encouraged me to find my 'happy place', which left me thinking… *What am I in for here?*

A young doctor came in and greeted us. He outlined what was to happen next and asked if I needed to hold his hand during the short procedure, mentioning the pain thing again. I reassured him that I was tough and I would be fine, but thanked him for his gesture. He paused, bunched up his lips and asked again. 'Are you sure?' The first nurse leaned in and whispered, 'It really hurts. Hold his hand, why don't you?' I flicked my eyes over to John, raised my eyebrows, turned back and asked the doctor, 'Do you *want* me to *want* to hold your hand?' Reaching over, he grabbed my hand and it was a done deal. The nurse asked me not to look. I took no notice. The small syringe housed a bright yellow substance making me all too aware that I was in the nuclear department of a hospital.

The doctor squeezed my hand in anticipation, but aside from the early sharp, scratch sensation, it was relatively pain-free. What an anticlimax! I smirked when I thought about the earlier drama in the room. Looking at me, the doctor asked if I was okay. I smiled and nodded. He turned to John and passed comment on the fact that he was married to a strong woman, very brave and stoic. John thanked him and laughed. I just took it all in my stride. The nurse told us that some women scream the place down and need lots of reassurance after the event. I was to have both breasts taken off permanently and tackle a mastectomy soon. There was no room for screaming over a small syringe. Not in my world.

The next morning was surgery day and my nerves had changed to excitement. It had been thirty-three days since the ultra-sonographer had spotted the 'speck' and I was ready. It was a strange feeling driving in the dark to the hospital to have cancer removed from my body when all around you the world is slowly awakening and other people's regular routines are simply ticking over. I thought about all those people getting up to go to work, the gym or having breakfast. The world was just getting on with it while I was about to start on operation number one.

However, it would turn out to be an enormous battle peppered with surgeries.

TIPS ABOUT WHAT TO PACK FOR THE HOSPITAL
- A journal – if writing is your way of expression, this is great to offload thoughts and feelings.
- Any questions you may have going into surgery that you have thought of between your last specialist meeting and your surgery.
- Health insurance details.
- Medicare card and any relevant medical records, pathology and scan results you have.
- Soft bra – I wore one as my scar went around my areola. Most women are advised to wear a comfortable, non-wired supportive bra following surgery.
- A good book or magazine to read.
- Lip balm for when you wake up from surgery.
- Slippers and comfortable bed socks.
- A LONG phone charger – not your usual standard-sized one.
- Dressing gown.
- Face wipes/ tissues and other toiletries you may require.
- Comfort blanket and your personal pillow (if you want to).
- Snacks. Mints are handy, especially after dry mouth!
- Water bottle – water jugs are supplied with polystyrene cups.
- Healthy snacks – your taste buds may be off-kilter from the surgery.

I checked in, was weighed, my vitals taken, hopped into a gown and began the wait. Not long after, I was taken downstairs into a very small room which had only the bed that I was on and an ultrasound machine. I was met by an elderly doctor who identified himself by his nickname. I loved this and felt at ease with a doctor with this habit and attitude towards his patients. I once taught a female child in Grade Four whose surname was Potter and I asked her permission to call her Harry for the rest of the year. She agreed and at the end of that academic year, she wrote to me full of thanks saying how she had really loved the nickname.

The pre-procedure I was to have before the lumpectomy is called wire localisation. I was given a local anaesthetic to the breast and then under ultrasound, the doctor was responsible for placing a titanium-based marker (a clip) directly into my tumour to make detection during the lumpectomy easier for my breast surgeon. It would also act as a guide to the precise area that was to be removed during my surgery. Sounds gross, right? This clip is at the end of the wire, similar to fishing line. While the clip was being inserted into the tumour, it was clear that the doctor was struggling. He passed comment that my tumour was 'solid' and I recoiled at the thought.

My breast surgeon appeared all smiles, greeted me and John, and we headed straight off for surgery. I kissed John goodbye and we parted ways with me calling out, 'I'm all good, John! I've got this!'

After I reached a small room connected to the theatre, the anaesthetist inserted a cannula in the back of my hand. It was remarked that my veins were nice and 'juicy' and the whole thing was relatively pain-free. I have never had any aversions to hospitals, blood work, needles or anything medical really, which, when you read on, you will realise is a good thing.

The operating theatre was full when I was rolled in. *All these people for a 'speck'*, I thought. The theatre was cold, very cold. There was also music playing and I inquired as to who selected the tracks for the sessions. They told me they took turns, but it had to be agreed by all. A nurse said they had never been asked that before and I wondered why. They all laughed and began a debate on the topic of who was selecting the next day's playlist.

I was ready. In this moment, cold and vulnerable, I decided I'd move forward with my life as quickly as possible after this nightmare was over. I knew early on that my recovery had to start from within. That cancerous mass did not deserve my attention, tears, or my worry; it was to have no power over me anymore. I felt a sense of 'being released' from cancer's grip that day – a feeling I'd craved over the last few weeks. I was in charge of my future mentally, just not necessarily physically, and I had to ride the wave of preventative medicine and treatments for a while.

I was still working hard to convince myself that this was just bad luck and nothing that I'd done. I still needed to fully understand and accept that cancer does not discriminate – ever. This was something that I struggled with for some time, being convinced it was something I had done. On that day, I hoped I would've enough future mental toughness to train my brain not to worry for the rest of my life. I had to not let cancer thoughts rule me or control me. I was in charge here, not it! Changing my inner dialogue had to happen because, if I'm truly honest, and as I was about to learn, I had to be rock solid in order to achieve this.

It was 'go' time. I was given a drug that made me slightly groggy. I caught a glimpse of my breast surgeon and thanked her. It may have been just another breast to her, just another day at the office, but this surgery for me was much, much more than that: it was life-saving. It would allow me to live long, grow old with John, and watch our children flourish. While answering the anaesthetist's questions and in a very short space of time, I found myself feeling very 'floaty'. I heard myself getting louder and fighting to get words out as I answered their questions. Falling deeper into the grip of the anaesthetic, I felt a mask being placed over my face and took some deep breaths. During those breaths, I just had time to wonder, *Where do you go when you are under?* Suddenly, I was gone. The lights were out.

I heard hushed tones first, followed by machines beeping and the soft squeak of shoes moving around the recovery room. A friendly-faced nurse with a bright-red hair net stroked my head and I was catapulted back to my childhood again. Her tone was calm and sweet. She promised to look after me until I was feeling well enough to go up to the ward. Remembering why I was here prompted me to feel a little emotional. I was emotional because it was over. I had waited a while to get to this place and the lumpectomy was finally done. The cancer was gone.

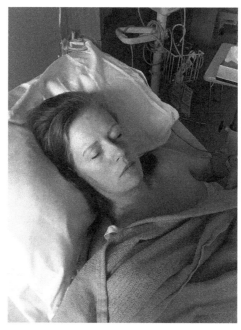

Recovering after my lumpectomy. February 2018.

I lifted my gown on the right and could see a small dressing over the left side of my right nipple. The difference in my breast size was immediately noticeable, but I didn't care. I was to have a mastectomy and knew things would even out. The next morning, I woke feeling new and happy. I was less groggy, and of course I had the satisfying feeling of being cancer-free. I recall a sense of relief that the stress of cancer choosing me was now over.

After staying in the hospital only one night and preparing myself for discharge, I noticed I had two dressings: the one on my right breast and one under my arm. My mind immediately shot to Sylvie, who had shown me a scar in her armpit because, at the time of her surgery, there was lymph node involvement. I felt desperate. *What were they looking for? What had they found?* I was comfortable that I had a brilliant breast surgeon, but my adrenalin kept rushing.

John arrived to take me home and I was told to leave the dressing on, keep it clean and not to do any heavy lifting. My wound would be checked and the results of the pathology would be discussed during my post-op appointment. I left feeling happy with my treatment by everyone at the hospital and was provided with enough information about how to manage once I got home. I accepted that I would have two scars instead of one and this did not bother me at all. Scarring has always fascinated me. With any operation, scarring is unavoidable. Scars carry stories.

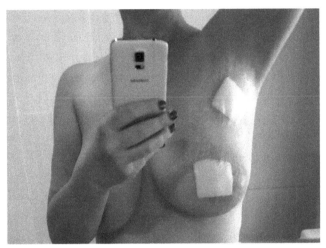

The following days post lumpectomy.
Note the Smurf style breast!

John and I attended my breast surgeon's private rooms seven days later to be met with the friendly nature of the secretary. The attitude of the 'front face' can really make a difference when you have multiple medical appointments. It can shape your mood and make everything seem okay when you feel the natural warmth of another human being. This day was one of those days. She managed to make me feel relaxed and cheery. However, my mood was about to be shattered.

My surgeon called us in and we exchanged pleasantries. Dissolvable stitches had been used for this surgery so I was expecting only a post-op check-up and to be told that my pathology was all clear (in keeping with my positive mindset).

She didn't mess around. Just like she did with my diagnosis, she got straight to it. She told us that, unfortunately, the tumour that I had was substantially larger than the ultrasound had picked up. It was four centimetres in size and this news now impacted the plan that we had in place. Three sentinel lymph nodes had also been removed and cancer had been found in one of them.

We were shattered and I was lost in my own thoughts for a moment. I thought about how this tumour had grown and gone undetected – for how long is anybody's guess – by the time it was found. It had leaked and spread out of my breast like lava from a volcano. The truth is that sometimes in life we *can* be unlucky. I was quiet, deflated, feeling ripped off and a little bit angry. I was dealing with so many emotions in that room. Reality bit. There was now some talk of maybe doing chemotherapy. Even mentioning this as an option really shocked me more than the diagnosis, because I wasn't expecting that word to be part of my cancer equation. It was going to be my choice if I wanted it or not and I was quickly referred to a Peninsula-based medical oncologist to discuss it further.

Eventually, we got around to removing the dressings from the surgery, revealing an incredibly neat lumpectomy scar around my areola and an equally neat one (about four centimetres under my arm). It wasn't deep in the armpit, just in that spot between the armpit and the breast. There was obvious blue dye in both areas and I was told it would be several weeks until that would go away. My urine was slightly blue and Layla cracked jokes about me being part Smurfette. With me, the dye lingered and was still there after many months.

Without dressings, my right breast remained noticeably smaller than the left, but that was the least of my worries. The new post-op plan was to have chemotherapy, which my oncologist would guide me through. Following this, I would have a breast reduction on one side to make the breasts even, then radiation therapy. The icing on my cancer cake was a double mastectomy later in the year. My wounds were redressed and I was sent home. We drove home with a small pillow between me and the seatbelt. Once again, my feelings were all over the place and my brain was in overdrive. I was scared – not for me, but for my family.

The following night, I sent out a group text asking friends and work colleagues to go and get a boob check, and urging them to let me know when they got the all-clear. Again this overwhelming sense of helping others get the all-clear consumed my thoughts. I wondered what it all meant.

A few days later, I felt very uncomfortable in my right armpit. I'm fairly tough so I ignored it for as long as I could, putting it down to the healing process, but it got to the point where I couldn't move without it being sensitive. On a more serious note, I couldn't lift the kettle to fill it with water for my tea! It felt like there was a golf ball in there. I began using my small bean-bag travel pillow to make it comfortable to even place my arm next to my body. There was also some visible swelling.

Not deeming it serious enough for the breast surgeon, I visited my local doctor, and he ordered a CT scan of the area. This revealed a large pocket of fluid that needed to be drained. I called my breast surgeon and she asked if I could come straight in to see her. This was no problem and I wondered if I should've done that in the first place. I made my way there and she told me it was called a seroma and needed to be drained (aspirated) with a needle under ultrasound. She could do it there and then.

As I hopped onto the bed, she took out a needle. Okay, when I say needle, I mean a NEEDLE. It was huge. Then she said the following, 'We won't need any anaesthetic because your scar will still be numb from the surgery.' WHAT? What on earth? In the needle went and my yoga breathing got a serious workout. It went very deep and when she pulled it out, she showed me. Surprisingly, it wasn't too bad at all. It was the idea of it that scared me. Bright orange fluid filled the syringe and she told me she would have to go in again as there was still more fluid in there. Yikes!

I was doing well over the next few weeks. My body felt strong but then familiarity came knocking. I began to experience similar feelings from when I had the seroma. Luckily, when I rang my surgeon straight away, she was in the breast clinic at the hospital on that particular day. I was home alone and the hospital was an hour away, forcing me to get a friend to drive me as I could not move my arm properly.

This was one of the first of many visits that would find me commuting up and down that same highway for months and months and months. At the same time, it would be the highway where I strengthened bonds with the various friends and family members who came to appointments to support me, so for that I'm grateful. Once there, the same deep penetrative procedure was carried out and thankfully, it never happened again.

A common and upsetting misconception is that once the cancer is excised, that's the end of it and all is well, but this could not be further from the truth. Even in my social setting, I got the feeling that some people were expecting that I was 'better' once I was free of the tumour. Yes, I was trying to put on a brave face, but at times I wasn't succeeding. Even a year on, I would continue to shower-cry in secret and endure feelings of despair at times for the 'old me' to return. Luckily, moments of weakness didn't last long and I would pull myself together and just charge forward. I had to continue to celebrate the tumour removal and recognise that it was quite easy and not at all as bad as I'd imagined.

Unusual and beautiful things in my everyday life started to happen. Strangers would contact me offering help. My school mums' group was amazing with school pick-ups and drop-offs so I could rest when I needed. Delicious home-cooked goodies once again lay on my front doormat.

There was even a time while shopping for some clothes, Lennox struck up a conversation with a shopkeeper with the result being him walking out with a few free items that made his day. Apparently, Lennox had been having a good old chat about his mum who was super brave and had cancer cut out of her body. The shopkeeper called me over, offering me a casual hat with a crown on the front. Lennox and I were delighted. We all embraced before we left and I promised to do a crown-hat selfie on my socials for her. She told me to 'be a queen'. I laughed, telling her that I was one already. It wasn't only that random act of kindness that made me feel so happy – Lennox was confident and comfortable enough to have a conversation with a stranger about what was going on in his world. I told him how proud I was of him as I tucked him into bed that night, and he said he was going to try it in the sweet shop next time. Clever little cookie!

I decided to use the power of social media with friends and family to raise awareness in and around the subject of breast cancer. I began by calling one of my lifelong friends, Damo, and he guided me through setting up a Facebook page called Rainbows & Sunflowers. This page had a profile picture sporting Roisin and me in happier times. It was taken when I travelled to the

U.K. for her thirtieth fancy dress birthday party. She was dressed as Barbie and I was dressed as Dame Edna. Looking back now, I revel in that photo. With no health problems in sight, we are simply loving life.

We love life now, but in a different way. A donations section was set up where our friends and family could support a reunion between me and Roisin once this nightmare was over. We were met with such generosity and warmth by people who empathised with us. From the outside, friends have told me it was an awful scenario for them as observers to be connected. One family, three out of six siblings struck by cancer, just needing to be together and have a great big hug, but bound by restriction. Believe me when I say, the prospect of a reunion with my unwell 'baby' sister lit my fire, propelling me forward and giving me extra 'grit' to fight as hard as I could.

Six

Choosing to swim

'I have learned over the years that when one's mind is made up, this diminishes fear; knowing what must be done does away with fear.'
Rosa Parks

I chose this.
Not everyone has chemotherapy.
Seeing myself as cancer's victim is not something I have ever entertained. Chemotherapy, to me, symbolised the next stage of my recovery, a necessary evil to help me keep cancer away, permanently. When I would encounter problems as a child, I would run to Mum with the problem written all over my face and she would always say, 'Well Lindsey, you can either sink or you can swim.'

Choosing to swim now, as an adult, is easy for me because I wasn't trying to stay alive just for me; it was all about John, Layla and Lennox. I was thrown into the eye of a storm, my reality upended in an attempt to stay alive and, even though my healing was going to be difficult to navigate, I promised myself to do it with a smile on my face.

Chemotherapy is the use of drugs that aim to destroy cancer cells in the body or to stop them from multiplying and spreading. The main purpose of my next meeting with my oncologist was to order a few tests and put a plan in place now that things for me had changed. She offered her sincerest apologies that we even had to meet under these circumstances, which I thought was lovely. It was disappointing news about cancer spreading out of the breast, but I was up for the fight. I knew that, typically, having chemotherapy could lower the risk of my breast cancer ever coming back. John and

I decided there and then that I would resign from work and take the rest of the year off. This was a decision that, had it not been made, would have been forced upon me anyway.

We went on to discuss different chemotherapy drugs. Unfortunately, I already knew about chemotherapy because I'd attended sessions with both my siblings. I was familiar with the fact that there were periods of recovery in between treatments; I knew about it being administered intravenously and its potency; and of course, I knew about the potential to endure dreadful side effects.

I told the oncologist that because of Roisin's second diagnosis, we had booked tickets to go to the U.K. to see our families. She bit the corner of her lip, suggesting that if we were to go ahead with chemotherapy plans, I wouldn't be able to take those flights. John and I asked to be excused for a moment. We stood outside in the fresh air and, after a brief discussion, we decided that John would take the trip along with our children and I would remain at home and stay with Mandy for a while. This was a deal I was completely comfortable with. I didn't *want* to have chemotherapy, but I chose this preventative measure for me and my family. I thought of our children and wanted to devote this 'time off' to giving it all I had. Cancer was only going to take a year off me, that's was all I was affording it. I was only going to get this once!

It wasn't until I had to walk into the travel agent's office to cancel my ticket that my emotions got the better of me. Cancelling my flight was unbelievably hard and I choked on the words. I went in, swallowed hard and did what I had to do. As I was walking away, I felt a lump in my throat and it broke me. I am from tough stock and not a big crier by nature (until cancer), but I was devastated, truly heartbroken. Heading straight to the closest public toilets, I locked myself in a stall and cried into my jacket. Chemotherapy would assist in this disease hopefully never coming back, so there was no question whether to have it or not, but that day, the decision to cancel my ticket came at a very high emotional price.

Bumping into some friends from John's old soccer club while shopping, I excused myself. Turning away, I could hear John filling them in about my cancer diagnosis. The sudden sting of tears caught me off guard, but I managed to fight them off. I despised the fact that John had to go through this. It was the age-old ripple effect. Yes, I got the disease, but it was impacting so many people around me. Sometimes I wondered if it affects those closest to the patient more than the person diagnosed. John was tough – really tough – and he'd handled everything so far with composure. He'd only briefly cried from worry on the day I found the lump and I knew he was being strong for all four of us.

We picked up some comfortable white bedding sets and lovely cushions that would no doubt be propping me up for the next few months as I headed towards 'destination chemotherapy'. I spoke to John about my 'near tear' incident as we left and he told me he was totally fine and to not worry about him. They left for England a few days later.

A chemotherapy education session was run by my local hospital before the commencement of my treatment. My lovely Mandy came along to act as that second set of ears. The session aimed to fully explain, in detail, everything there was to know about what would be happening to me over the next three months. This session also outlined the potential side effects of what chemotherapy could do to my body, but not necessarily what it would do.

Over the next three months, chemotherapy had the potential to compromise my immune system, lower my red blood cells, probably constipate me and affect my oral health. I was supplied with dental mouthwash and toothpaste to avoid cottonmouth. Mouth ulcers were common, as well as a very strange metallic taste in the mouth. It might also lift my nails and maybe make me sick. Hair loss would definitely happen, as it was the number one side effect of the drug I was scheduled to have first – docetaxel. Nausea would almost certainly come knocking, but would be sent marching with powerful anti-nausea medication made available to me.

I needed my armour to be thick and I found that every conversation with my sister helped. Talking it through with her calmed me every time. Hot flushes or night sweats could happen, fatigue could set in, nails could fall off, bone density could be compromised, not to forget the possible 'chemo fog'. Had I made the right decision to undertake this step? Of course I had. I remembered the alternative.

Providing me with a medical alert notification card allowed me to be seen immediately in the Emergency Department, in the case of a rise in my body temperature. If it rose to 37.5, I was to present at the E.R. straight away.

One thing I decided to do was to attend my chemotherapy sessions looking sharp. Having some control made me feel better. Roisin told me she put on her best dress complete with a full face of make-up, and it made her feel so much better on the day. So, that is what I did. Putting a picture of myself on my social media page after the session was a given, so it made sense really. Super vain I know, but if you've got it, flaunt it, right?

Following the information overload session at the hospital, Mandy invited me for dinner that night so I could relay the information to John accurately, with her filling in the missing parts. What a friendship! The education session took about two hours altogether. I was weighed and measured on that day so they had a baseline about my health and it concluded with being given a tour of the unit. It was smaller than I expected, with the chairs lined around the perimeter of the ward filled with patients eating, knitting, chatting and sleeping. Gentle waves and small smiles were cast in my direction from patients and I imagined myself in their shoes in a short week's time.

On the way out, one of the flyers from the education session caught my eye. It was for 'Mummy's Wish', a not-for-profit charity that's been in operation for ten years. Their mission is to support Australian families with children aged twelve years and under whose mum has been affected by cancer. Calling them was a wise choice as I received such wonderful support. Within a few days, our children had a parcel in the post addressed to them with a 'Mummy's Wish' label on it. After the five long minutes Layla and Lennox spent playing 'Rock, Paper, Scissors' to decide who was going to open it, they were snuggling the softest brown bears you could ever want.

Inside the bears were heart-shaped voice recorders on which anyone (mostly the patient) could leave a message. These teddies became instant hits and cosy sleeping partners, and the voice recorders were the subject of lots of laughs over the coming months – they even once appeared at school in the kids' lunchboxes. They loved them. Messages of encouragement recorded on them by friends of mine were a treat too and their smiles said it all. Later on in the year, the charity also provided some nutritious family meals to help out, which were greatly appreciated. Even though I was capable of cooking for my family, this certainly lightened my load.

Before chemotherapy, I had an important job to do. I had to hand back my work key for the school from which I had just resigned. I arranged to travel to Mornington to meet Naomi at one of our favourite cafés. She brought her six year-old daughter Lily along to chat with me. Tears welled in Naomi's eyes when I pulled out the key. That key opened the door to my second home. We both loved our jobs – she had been 'my person' there and vice versa. That key brought us together. That key let us in the building to cheer each other up if the chips were down.

At that moment, in that café, on that day, we dared not speak because if we did, those tears that were teetering on falling would surely not stop for a while. So we didn't. We just embraced. Poor Lily was left playing head tennis and wondering what was going on as two fully grown women were silently nodding, hugging, slightly crying in the middle of the day, all with a key in the middle of us.

Early April saw a bone scan at the request of the oncologist. It required an injection beforehand and was administered to detect fractures, cancer, infections and other abnormalities in my bones. Mandy's daughter, Fay, tagged along to keep me company as I had to lie under the scanner for forty-five minutes. It was such a relief to read, 'This is a negative study for osteoblastic metastatic activity'.

I nicknamed one of my handbags 'the chemo bag'. I found myself constantly surprised by how many items I could fit in there. It mimicked a magician's hat. In fact, I had so much in there, John remarked that I looked like I was off to the pamper salon. That was it! After that remark, I treated my chemotherapy sessions as just that. Time for me… downtime. Maybe I should have packed my fluffy slippers?

THINGS I BROUGHT TO CHEMOTHERAPY SESSIONS:
- Support partner – who also doubled as a taxi driver.
- Sick bag – just in case, you don't want to upset your driver!
- Book of positive affirmations/cards.
- Good book.

- Phone charger/iPod/laptop – make yourself a playlist, download some podcasts, use your laptop to catch up on emails of friends who have contacted you or to keep family updated.
- Crosswords/Sudoku/puzzle books to keep your mind sharp.
- Headphones – I had noise-cancelling ones.
- Blanket – I used the one Cindy and Damo had bought for me as it made me feel close to them.
- Ask for ice chips – they can help with mouth sores.
- Tissues – sometimes your nose can run if you lose your nose hair!
- Travel cup for my tea – I packed my own caffeine-free tea bags.
- Bottle of water – glass.
- Lip balm.
- Healthy snacks – they do offer you something light.
- Possibly slippers?? It could feel like you are at home or having a day at the spa!

It may seem like a long list of items but one of my nicknames is 'safety girl'. I'm a 'just in case' kind of packer which stems from my years of camping.

While having chemotherapy was nothing to laugh about, a sense of humour was required about now, as well as a heart full of gratitude. Using self-talk and thinking that there were people in the world worse off than I was helped during my 'blue moments'. I had to train my mind not to get caught up in my feelings – not to dwell. Negative thoughts were locked out, not allowed in, not capable of altering my mindset, not on those difficult days.

Eventually, it was time for John, Layla and Lennox to return from the U.K. and I was excited. I'd put in a rather large request of all the British treats that I liked and missed. Being a lady of leisure had been so relaxing while they were away but I really couldn't wait to see them all. I was especially proud of my Layla. While in the U.K., Roisin had taken her to a hair salon to cut off her long, brown, curly hair to donate it to charity. Proud is an understatement!

The day before my chemotherapy commenced, I had to have bloodwork done. This was to determine that I was well enough to manage the chemo. Working full-time, dashing to our children's after-school activities and running the house changed to constant appointments and tedious glossy magazine-flicking in waiting rooms which became my new 'normal'.

I had walked past the chemotherapy unit door at my local hospital so many times and had always offered a silent prayer for the patients there. This was because I'd watched so many people in my family struggle with cancer. My heart went out to them and I wished them well, never once thinking that I would be one of them myself. Walking into the chemotherapy unit on day one, I thought, *Things will be back to normal soon, I'm sure.*

Seven

Chemical blur

*'The job of chemotherapy would be to cut off my cancer's food supply.
It was not going to get me. I was going to starve it to death.'*
Josepha Dietrich-cancer survivor

Day one was finally here. I felt strong, but tentative. I had been given a medicine in tablet form that was to be taken the night before chemo- therapy sessions and for two days post-therapy at the same time. It was called dexamethasone – a steroid medication to minimise nausea – and I had to record it on a provided chart. On that same chart was a list of side effects which I had to tick. This was so I could be closely monitored and deal with any of them swiftly. Even though the oncologist wouldn't let me suffer, I wasn't about to become a hero.

Being a steroid-based drug meant there were a few bodybuilding jokes thrown around by my friends as a joke, but muscles never happened. In fact, the opposite happened. The chemotherapy medication did nothing but inflate me like a balloon, and it was to be a long time before I could even contemplate regaining my normal weight. I bloated, and very quickly. It didn't take long before I resembled Violet Beauregarde from *Charlie and the Chocolate Factory*. Dexamethasone also made my scalp itch, really itch. I even got scalp pimples from as early as day three!

I was also putting on weight, and fast. What was worse, chemotherapy dosages are worked out according to weight. Therefore, as I grew, I would have to manage more of the damn medication. When I tried to make light of my new Violet Beauregarde-look, people would be kind and say, 'Don't be silly', or 'Don't worry about how you look now. Worry about that later'. But deep down, it was all about control for me. I had to learn to embrace my curves, otherwise I was going to get depressed. At times, it was sad looking at my unwell reflection during the treatment period, but, again, I rationalised it by holding onto the fact that it was only going to be temporary.

In the infusion area of the chemotherapy ward above the chairs, there were TVs which nobody watched. I checked in on my mindfulness as I sat in the oversized armchair and I was surprisingly calm. Was it because I was too familiar with the regimen of chemotherapy or was it because I had fantastic support from John? Probably a bit of both. The only worry I had was about vomiting. I have never been a person who vomits. I just can't deal with it. The whole idea of food returning after being in my body for many hours disgusts me.

My eyes swept the room and it became apparent that I was the youngest. History was repeating itself. This had happened to my brother, Sean, my sister, Roisin, and now me. I was the youngest in many of the waiting rooms in which I sat during my illness and it always left me feeling pissed off.

Round one of four began. The nurse talked me through the process of what she was going to do and what would happen if I had an allergic reaction. The whole process of getting ready took around half an hour. Most of that was because we had to wait for my bags of chemotherapy to arrive on the ward fresh from the 'chemo warehouse'. The nurse began work setting up. First she had to cannulate the back of my hand and then she administered the drugs intravenously, starting with saline followed by docetaxel, saline again followed by drug number two, cyclophos-phamide. Each bag took around thirty minutes to empty, with the bags being on an intravenous pole which allowed me to move freely around the room.

One great photograph taken is of my sister during her chemotherapy, where she is wheeling her drip to the bathroom, then pauses to kiss the pole. I wondered why? Was she as grateful as I was to know there is medicine that gave us the best possible chance of removing the leftover dodgy cells in our bodies? I felt lucky to be in the public system once again, especially after hearing the price of a single bag of chemo, and I was having two of them!

Physically feeling the fluid go into my arm (or anywhere else actually) never happened. It was a relief knowing that the chemotherapy in those moments was acting as the silent slayer of cancer cells.

Each chemotherapy treatment is personalised depending on the cancer type, cancer stage, and body weight. My drug cocktails took between two-and-a-half and three hours all up, during which time I chatted with John. Thank goodness some chemotherapy days fell on his rostered days off. He was great at seeing life from a different perspective from mine and even better at managing any worries I may have had.

The ward was noticeably quiet. The nurse came and chatted with me, which gave John licence to quietly nod off or grab some lunch from the café. I ran the idea past the nurse of starting an initiative on the topic of checking your breasts regularly and general breast health. She agreed with the need to educate people more, and as an educator, I knew I had to make some noise about this subject! Talking about your 'bits' can be embarrassing and often viewed as taboo – after all, they are called private parts – but I felt strongly about this and these thoughts weren't going away.

Following chemotherapy and over lunch with John, I got the giggles. I felt slightly drunk and was speaking about random topics quite uncharacteristically. It was a happy day and I was comfortable realising that I was a quarter of the way through my chemotherapy.

Home found me resting in my 'chemo chair'. Chemotherapy fatigue is so different from regular fatigue. Previously, I would get tired only at bedtime, which, in my 'old life', was eleven o'clock, but this felt different. One suggestion that is echoed throughout all the cancer organisations is that exercise aids healing and helps fatigue. I know it sounds counterintuitive, but it is true. Releasing endorphins seemed common sense, yet here I was spending a lot of time sitting in the 'chemo chair' ironically watching re-runs of *Grey's Anatomy* on television with just enough energy to walk the dog. This was a non-negotiable, by the way. I would've had the 'evil mother' death stare from our Maltese Shih-Tzu, Melfi, if I didn't!

Chemotherapy kills anything that has fast-growing cells. Over time, I noticed the lining of my mouth changing. Placing my finger in my mouth and sweeping the inside of my cheek meant that I'd see pieces of my skin on my finger, like tiny pink ball bearings. The inside of my mouth was literally falling off! Then came the metallic taste. Overall, that taste and the mouth ulcers were just plain annoying.

Additionally, the taste and the texture of food completely changed only a few days post-treatment. I recall eating a cracker, hearing the crunch and thinking I was eating cardboard. As my tastebuds changed, everything became increasingly tasteless. As a foodie, this was hell. I even struggled to taste my cups of tea, which to me, was sinful. I was smiling at food gifts being delivered, knowing that only my family would reap the benefit of the culinary delights before me. I dismissed the idea of using any metal utensils and even went to Ikea to purchase plastic picnic cutlery – another Roisin tip. The only foods I could honestly taste were oranges and curries. I couldn't even taste the food required to assist in the constipation department – prunes, prunes and prunes. Did I mention prunes? I had quite a few poo pity parties in my bathroom during my treatment and took to reading in there, which horrified our children!

I had to self-administer an injection every second day for a short period after receiving chemotherapy. The injection was called Neulasta which stim- ulates the growth of white blood cells. It was going to support me against infection during this fragile time and it was to be kept in the fridge. It offended me every time I opened the fridge to see the hospital esky filled with needles next to delicious food that I couldn't taste.

As chemotherapy medication is toxic, it can make others sick if they come into contact with it, so precautions had to be taken. I was informed that my family could share the same bathroom with me, but only if I flushed twice after a powder room visit for at least two days and wiped down the toilet with antiseptic wipes. No flushing those, of course. I didn't want any turtles choking to death. The reason for the extra precaution is because the chemicals are still in the body for around forty-eight hours post-treatment and it could have made John or the children unwell.

I also had a separate face washer, hand towel and bath towel, with abso- lutely no sharing. I upped the frequency of hand sanitiser and even kept some by the front door for visitors with a very clear message: 'Welcome, now be cleansed!' It was suggested that if any sexual relations were to take place, which was hardly ever as I had the libido of a corpse (another cancer gift), then we were to use condoms.

Infusion leads to confusion! My mental dexterity was being compromised. Dexamethasone, or 'the dreaded dexa' as I soon nicknamed it, gave me insomnia for about four days after each dose. However, I favoured this over nausea any day of the week. Insomnia was long-term for me and probably the most irritating side effect during my treatment. It confused my body and disorganised my thoughts. I tried making the connection to cognitive change – you know the proverbial 'chemo brain' or 'chemo fog' directly linked to lack of sleep – but later on (okay, even present-day), I realised that it was just a lack of brain cells on my part because I was so tired.

One disturbing day, I was driving to the hospital and found myself sitting at a familiar intersection. I knew this road like the back of my hand, yet I could not decide to turn left or right. I was stuck. Why could I not make a decision right or left? How could this be? Later, relaying the incident of that morning made me cry for ages all over John's t-shirt.

My brain was behaving very strangely indeed. I wanted an envelope but asked for a stamp. Everything turned into a 'whatdoyacallit' and a 'thingy-majig'. If I was trying to remember the name of a friend, not necessarily a close friend, I could tell you everything about them with their name on the tip of my tongue, but I could not get their name out of my mouth. I'm embarrassed to say this but I found myself on more than one occasion having to search social media so their photograph would trigger my memory. I was so happy to be temporarily out of the workplace as I seriously felt too dumb to return. Frustrated at all the errors I was making gave me an unfamiliar feeling of inadequacy. There were only three days in a three-week chemotherapy cycle where I had utter fatigue, and for that, I was grateful. However, the chemo fog remained staunch.

My oncologist did everything to ensure I was as comfortable as possible during treatment, but I was responsible for managing my emotional state. Diffusing my trusty lavender essential oil and drinking sleepy tea potions from my friend, Aliesha – 'the little blonde naturopath' (her cool business name) – helped me because tea heals everything, right? I also got some apps on my phone and entered into the world of meditation. Even though

I couldn't sleep for most of the night, I wasn't too worried as I felt relaxed by tapping into my spiritual side, which was not very spiritual back then, I assure you!

The bonus of insomnia was that my U.K.-based family were all awake, so I worked out all their days off and chatted endlessly, connecting with them on a deeper level. My siblings have always been a fun bunch all my life. Terrence (oh dear, that's so formal) – Terry – is the firstborn in the family and came into this world a mere thirteen months before me. We had to wait six years before we had a sibling with whom to play, so our bonds as toddlers and then school-aged children were well and truly solid. Terry lives in England with his wife, Claire, three children and young grandchildren. He would do anything for me, anything at all. He is someone you could call on in the middle of the night and he would fix whatever needed fixing.

While there was an abundance of sleeping aids out there, I never relied on anything pharmaceutical to aid sleep. I wanted to stay as clean as possible as I was already turning into Toxic Tina and fast!

Nail damage or nail loss was also on my gift-giving list from cancer. Most of my nails turned dark, loosened, and were pretty painful during the months of chemotherapy. I lost four toenails in total, which have grown back unusually stained. My hands were not too bad. They just look different from my 'old' nails and are extremely brittle, but nothing really to complain about. Chemo is so harsh on the body and mind overall. While painting my nails black made me feel 'gothic' and a need to switch on some Marilyn Manson tunes, I don't know if it helped at all because the reality is that chemotherapy was attacking me on a cellular level. During that ride, I just had to grab onto the sides and hope I made it out of there.

As toxic time began, I started to think about a fundraiser for when I lost my hair. I'd never had a big birthday celebration before – travelling fantastic parts of the earth had replaced boozy celebrations. Highlights included eating barbecued octopus in Santorini, riding camels on Christmas day in Cairo, and rafting down a river in Thailand. I promised myself that I would get better soon and enjoy more discovering. It was a 'life's too short' moment, and a moment on which I needed to act.

The Little Things

It was on a girl's weekend in the city with Mandy, filled with shopping and a little champagne, that we planned the head-shave fundraiser, and I knew it would be so much fun. For some, losing hair from chemotherapy is as bad as the cancer diagnosis itself. For me, it was a gateway to survivorship and I upheld the attitude of, *It's only hair*. It was decided that Mandy would host a 'Rainbows & Sunflowers' themed high tea in her back garden. I wanted to shave my head before it came out in clumps. I just wanted the control that came with getting there first. Cancer had recently been good at taking away some of my choices and I wanted to be the victor for once.

Twelve days after my first round of chemo, I woke up early and felt a hair in my mouth. I knew that baldness wasn't far away. I was born with deep red hair. You know the type – the type that gives licence to schoolyard bullies to call you names day after day, unable to think of anything nice to say. Gingernut, Duracell (Copper Coloured Top) and Carrot Top were popular. Back then, I could've cried, fought or even been scarred long-term from the verbal taunts but I didn't and I wasn't. Not only did I have the security of four brothers behind me, I also had no fear. In fact, I used to smile at them. I figured if you smile at someone being mean to you during the primary school taunts, they might just think you are crazy and leave you alone.

When I moved to Australia in 1997, I had a Nicole Kidman *Top Gun* hairstyle. At the time of treatment, my hair sat just below my shoulders and was glittered with white hair that matched my age. A streak that made me resemble Cruella De Ville appeared at the front of my head just after my fortieth birthday.

In the shower I noticed that I could pull out five or six hairs without any pain whatsoever, confirming 'it' was beginning. I did it again and it felt like a strange addiction. It was a beautiful afternoon in late April when we gathered for the head shave. John had donned a 'skinhead' type look for a few years now and we decided that he'd be the one to take the clippers to my head. People arrived from everywhere: the city, the hills, the peninsula and the suburbs. I had many friends from different social settings and we all came together for a great cause.

After some time, a stool was placed in the centre of the outdoor decking and butterflies were going crackers in my stomach. I could see a look of sadness in John's eyes. We shared a kiss and I told him once again, 'It's only hair'. I was witnessing his pain firsthand. Flanked by Layla and Lennox, we decided to tie my hair back in a loose ponytail first to make cutting it off easier. I'd chosen the song *I am Woman* by Australian icon Helen Reddy to play as my head was shaved, and we enjoyed hearing the lyrics blast all over the street that day:

'You can bend but never break me, 'cos it only serves to make me more determined to achieve my final goal. And I come back even stronger...'

John took a deep breath: *snip,* my ponytail was no more. It was like the scene from the movie 'Tangled' where, when her hair is cut, it dies. I looked down and didn't recognise it. The ponytail looked brown. It looked dead. When the first buzz of the clippers sounded, it was met with the supportive claps and cheers of my loved ones. No going back now, it was game on!

Perched on a stool, I looked down over the crowd of friends and family who were in the sunken garden and I beamed. I didn't cry, but I could see tears falling and rolling down cheeks dotted before me. Layla and Lennox were helping John by excitedly catching the hair as it fell. It didn't take long to complete and I was immediately complimented by the crowd about how much I suited my new convict look. I apparently have a nice-shaped head, something I had told my sister – twice. I held it together until I saw my friend, Luci. We embraced and then I cried, just a little, not for the hair loss but for the pain that cancer had caused those close to me.

I worked the room thanking my guests for their kind donations and felt amazingly liberated. At the high tea, people were donating money for two reasons: to offer some to charity, but also to help pay for a reunion between me and Roisin. When this rubbish was over, we desperately wanted to hug each other tightly. Little did I know, the way it all turned out was to be the biggest surprise of my life!

I relished in the amount of money I was going to save on haircuts, hair ties, and hair products, and delighted in the fact that I would save on hair washing, drying and straightening. Yes, I was good at finding silver linings that day. I became excited about how I could maybe turn my scarves into beautiful headwear and knew that all my beanies and hats would get a royal workout over my son's soccer season this coming winter.

Lennox was later to tell me a story of when he was playing a game one Saturday morning, there was a silhouette of a mother approaching the soccer pitch. One of his buddies asked him, 'Is that my mum?' He had replied, 'No, it's mine. I know it's her because she's had breast cancer and wears hats all the time now.' I loved the fact that he used the word, 'had'. Later that afternoon, John snapped a picture of me after the shave wearing a white beanie that was gifted to me. This photo later appeared in my local paper with an article on breast awareness.

At the close of the head shave, Layla gave a speech on my behalf. She was amazing and wooed the crowd. John quietly cried. The impact, once again, was so visible.

LAYLA:

'Mum asked me to speak on her behalf today for two reasons: one, because she thinks I'm capable enough, and two, because she can't guarantee she won't cry. Thank you, everyone, for coming today. Mum's diagnosis has been tough, given the circumstances with her sister and our aunty, but she's doing okay. On January 25th, when the ultrasound found the tumour, she thought about this day. She thought about how weird it was going to be to look like my dad, Lennox, her dad and her brothers. She thought about how she didn't have the ears for chemo! 'Like a taxi going down the street with its doors open,' her brothers used to tease. Anyway, we are here all together now and it's done, Mum. Thank you to Mandy, Rich and Fay for hosting. It is a great house for parties and somewhere Mum has always been welcome and felt at home. Mandy, my mum thinks you are a legend and is grateful for all the decorations and effort today. Thanks for all the food

that everyone has made or bought and brought along today to share. Thanks for always checking in on our mum and, most of all, thanks for the door fee donations. A large portion of that will go to the McGrath Foundation, which raises money to place nurses in cancer patients' homes. Did you know that men can get breast cancer too? You might not think about it, but they can... Lennox said, 'in their man boobs!!' My mum wants everyone to go home and 'Check your boobs, people!!' Once again, thanks to everyone. With love from The Kennedys.'

Over the next week, I would find short hairs EVERYWHERE: in my car, on my pillow, in my hats *and* in my tea! But back to later that night, when we shaved my head down to a number one buzz cut. It felt strange to think it'd be some time before hair would be growing back. We made a video and put it on our social media page, 'Rainbows & Sunflowers.' I wanted to offer bravery and strength to other women out there who will lose their hair, because for some this is traumatic. In the video, John is having some fun and gives me a 'Travis Bickle' haircut (the fictional protagonist from the 1976 movie, *Taxi Driver*).

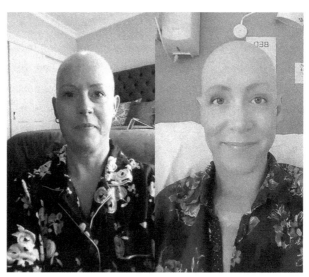

*Roisin and I 'twinning' as baldies during
our chemotherapy treatments.*

All the time, I would catch glimpses of myself in the kitchen's mirrored splashback and think, *Who the hell is that?* Lennox would rub my head and keep tabs on the regrowth! After a while, my head became very dry and I was feeling a sense of numbness too. Using lots of moisturiser was the key. It was a strange sensation, and once again, I put it down to the medicine. When in doubt, I would blame the chemical dump that was happening to me.

Following the head-shave a friend of ours, Johnny, contacted the major Australian television network, Channel 7. The producer called and put me onto the health reporter. They wanted to do a short piece for the news all about Roisin's and my story. It was the school holidays and Layla and Lennox were unbelievably excited at the idea of a news van parked outside, beaming our family story to the whole of Australia. While it was a good humanitarian piece, I was also excited at the prospect of expressing how important it was to be breast health aware.

The reporting team arrived, led by Georgia Main. The camera operator knew what he was after. Having tidied the whole house and purchased some beautiful fresh flowers, I was pleased to see him setting up in a nice nook of the house. Towards the end of filming, Lennox made us all laugh. Our dog, Melfi, had snuggled up to him and he stared into the dog's eyes exclaiming, 'Oh Melfi, I hope *you* don't get cancer'. That kid is a crack-up! Shortly after, Georgia said she could've chatted with me all day and that I had some vitally important things to say. It was on that day that I thought seriously about writing this book. Did I have the ability to be influential, even in the smallest capacity? I decided that I hadn't been given this motor mouth, good manners and confidence for nothing. I had a plan.

In the next shot, we were asked to make a video-call to my sister. We were having a good laugh about the time difference and how she'd had to get up at three in the morning, yet she still managed to look fantastic. She had been the one into make-up when we were growing up, always experimenting with colour and design. She was also very adventurous and creative and always looked so respectable.

After the news crew finished, the camera guy let the children play with the huge Channel 7 microphone. They loved pretending to be reporters and fake interviewing each other. I relished the moment – watching the kids so happy was lovely to see and it was happening more and more often lately. The news crew left, letting us know that they'd be back to film the reunion we so desperately wanted and that we'd be on the four and six o'clock news. How exciting! Glancing at the clock, I realised it was already three o'clock. I called my sister back and thanked her for the effort. As promised, we appeared on the news.

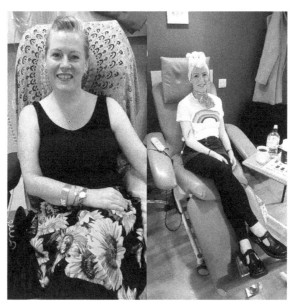

*Myself in Melbourne, Australia having chemotherapy
whilst Roisin is sat in Chorley, England.
May 2018*

The news story was fabulous. Just short of two minutes, it showcased that even though my sister and I were so many miles apart, we still managed to support each other wholeheartedly and how we had vowed to see each other again soon. It outlined our mission to not only raise awareness, but to help people realise how easy it is to raise much-needed funds for charity. I felt very proud and hoped that one day they would capture what would be the reunion of the century in our family life. Our mobile phones were pinging all night with only the kindest of words and encouragement for us.

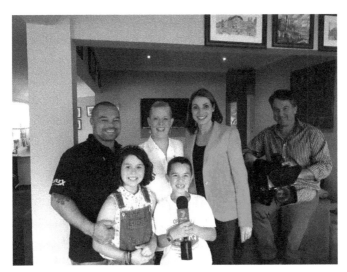

All of us with Georgia Main. Lennox
pretending to be a newsreader!

I remained on a high for the evening, but that night when I tried to sleep, I couldn't. I watched John sleep and hoped that we would grow old together. Left, right, left, right – there it was again. I had developed this rather pendulous behaviour of feeling great one moment and then questioning life the next. I was certainly behaving differently.

Not long after, I visited a bookstore, where the owner had told me that both she and her daughter, Nicole, had suffered breast cancer. She arranged for Nicole and me to meet up. Strangers helping strangers brought me pure joy. We met at my place and had an instant connection. She was so wonderfully optimistic and gave me some sound advice about wigs (for free), where to go to find them and how to wash them. She encouraged me to sleep on a silk or satin pillow as there would be less friction because, at times my shaved head resembled Velcro and was quite painful to the touch. Her knowledge and support were undeniable and I sat in awe of how the universe works.

Nicole directed me to a very professional charity called Think Pink. With a focus on wellness, not illness, Think Pink's Living Centre has a mission to provide practical support to both men and women, offering multiple opportunities to enable an easier journey for patients and their families. Connecting with them was wonderful. They offered me a one-to-one wig consultation and fitting, the opportunity to meet new friends facing similar battles, free massages, and days of indulgence where I could just relax. The best part was that it was all run by highly-trained breast care nurses whom I had access to anytime. John was also catered for. He attended a course called 'Supporting Blokes' and came back armed with both valid and relevant information for our situation. I am forever indebted to them because they stepped up to assist me at a very vulnerable time.

Slowly over time, I lost all of my body hair. Even my nose hair fell out, which led to some nosebleeds and a need to keep tissues in every jacket pocket I owned. The upside? Both my legs and armpits celebrated in unison.

Venturing out in public rocking the bald look was not high on my agenda. I could see other women who did and I smiled for them, but for me, even with my copious amounts of confidence, this would have crushed me. There is a fine line between nosiness and curiosity. Having cancer or wearing headwear associated with cancer can make you a target and strangers talking about it to you could go either way. It could either offend because, to be frank, we work bloody hard to stop thinking about it each day, or it could be used as an opportunity to be open and talk about it.

Being passionate and driven about raising awareness about checking yourself regularly was important to me, so I was an open book when it came to talking with strangers about it. In saying that, some people have no filters, like the time someone said to me, again in the supermarket, 'Having cancer must be horrible.' Yep, lady. It is! Lennox suggested I should've coughed loudly and told her if she got too close she could catch it. The children decided that next time, as a practical joke, I should wear a pink face mask that my Mum had sent me, then people would *really* back off for fear of contamination.

It was winter season during my treatment, so wearing beanies all day every day was not only comfortable but meant that I didn't have to explain myself to people all the time. The following month, I was invited to attend a course called, 'Look Good, Feel Better', courtesy of The Bays Hospital, Mornington, where my support group was held. It's a free initiative for men, women and teens run by volunteers. It is dedicated to teaching cancer patients how to manage the appearance-related side effects caused by cancer treatment. I had no hair and a history of being highly unsuccessful with make-up application, so I was sold! I entered the room with excitement, and once again, noticed I was the youngest in the room. I felt out of place but grateful for the opportunity at the same time. It was a workshop-style session and the staff was welcoming and friendly. I was wearing a pink head-scarf that tied at one side of my head and I knew that to get the most out of the skincare session, I had to remove it.

I had not done this yet in front of anyone but John, Layla and Lennox. I was unusually nervous and could feel my heart rate knocking furiously against my ribcage. There were so many occasions where I wanted to rock the bald look, sit in a café and be brave, but I never did. I removed the scarf slowly and realised that we were all in the same boat. My eyes swept the room and it was apparent that we were all at similar stages in our treatment. I sat down with a placemat and mirror in front of me, and before me lay a variety of make-up necessary to glam me up. I wondered how four volunteers were going to get around such a big group as time was limited. Then it hit me – I was to do my own. Gulp! I must admit I was rubbish at the make-up part. I just looked like I had been punched. It wasn't pretty. I had a few laughs at my own expense and had fun being a model for different head wraps and fringes. We all left feeling pretty damn special with a complimentary show-bag filled with skincare and make-up products donated by various cosmetic giants.

During the months I was having chemotherapy, my world shrunk, the time had simply disappeared and it had felt strange putting me first all the time. I had been a mother at that point for a decade and loved handing part of myself over to the children – not fully, because I understood that to be the best wife and mother I could, I also had to look after me, but this was different.

Over in the U.K., Roisin was a tiny step ahead of me. She had just finished her chemotherapy and there was an option to ring a bell. She rang the hell out of that thing. I didn't have a bell, so finishing my chemotherapy was rather boring. I was ready to shout from the rooftops if I'm honest, but I just felt tired and sad. Naomi reminded me that I didn't have to be strong ALL the time, which was timely advice. After my chemotherapy, naively, I thought I was well on the way to being cured – a word I found out later was rarely used in the cancer world.

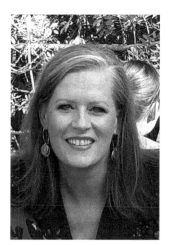
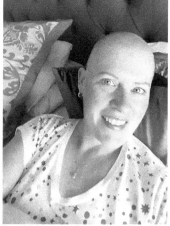

My strawberry blonde hair lost to chemotherapy. "It's only hair".

Eight

The Perfectionist

*'I have to say thank you. I found a lump in my breast after listening
to the 'Feel The Boobs' song. I had a mammogram, ultrasound
and a biopsy on Monday and I get my results soon. The doctor
said if it was indeed cancerous then it's small and very treatable.
It's now being dealt with and I'm very grateful to you all.'*
Joanne Evans – cancer patient

There it was, right there. Impact.

Having a positive impact or influencing someone else's life is something to be appreciated. Roisin and Michael had decided to re-write the lyrics from the very famous *Feed The World* song by Band Aid from 1984, re-naming it *Feel The Boobs*. Band Aid was a supergroup put together by Sir Bob Geldof in response to the famine that hit Ethiopia, 1983-1985. Sporting her new wig and surrounded by her friends one night, Roisin starred in an internet hit!

The revised lyrics read: (feel free to hum along as you read)

At shower time, there's no need to be afraid,
At shower time, have a feel, it'll be okay,
'Cos in this world of cancer, we can spread the word to all,
Check your boobs for lumps and bumps and cop a feel.
Yes, check your boob, then check the other one.
If there's a change, it's hard, but ring your doctor up.
There's a world of cancer treatments.

If caught early, you'll get the all-clear.
Our NHS is so amazing, nurses and docs are here.
And the fear will keep on ringing, and the clanging chimes of doom.
But tonight just have a shower and check your boobs.
And there won't be much to feel for most of the time.
But if you get a dimple, lump or rash,
Ohhhhh, well don't leave it to grow
Get it checked and don't be slow.
Do you know it's booby time at all?
Here's to boobs, cop a feel for everyone.
Yay for checks, don't forget your underarm.
Do you know it's booby time at all?
Feel the boooobs x 3
Let men know they get it too, and
Feel your boooobs.
Let them know it's booby time and
Feel the boooobs…

Because of that song, a magical moment – albeit brief – happened. On the night of the recording, my sister video-called, directing me to pin my hair up and apply bright lipstick because she wanted me to join in a fun song she was recording. I got to work. It took me three attempts singing into my mobile phone, but I finally sent her a one-line video with which I was pleased. I then had serious giggles sending her all my earlier bloopers!

My line: **'Let them know it's booby time and'**…
Feel the boooobs
Let them know its booby time x 3
Feel the boooobs, let them know it's booby time tonight!

The song was a huge success. A media company picked it up and wrote an article about sisters battling cancer on opposite sides of the world who had made a *Feel The Boobs* song to raise funds. It was one of those times in life when you reflect and it makes you smile. I was once again gushy proud of my baby sister.

Later that month, I received a text message from Roisin. A woman by the name of Joanne had contacted her after hearing the song. She was writing a letter of thanks for the awareness raised about the importance of self-checking. She'd followed the directives of the catchy song's lyrics, and there it sat – a small but obvious lump in her breast. A follow-up with her G.P. revealed she had in fact developed early stage breast cancer which, luckily, was very treatable. She was thrilled and so pleased that there were people such as us out there who cared for others. What a first-class feeling! It was utterly brilliant and Roisin and I agreed that it was one of the best feelings we'd ever experienced in our lives.

Roisin's song was the difference between an early-stage and a too-late-stage diagnosis and we were all privileged to be a tiny part of that.

In my everyday conversations, I chat with everyone about breast cancer, but only if the timing is right. I consider it my form of paying it forward. I don't force the topic onto people, but if it comes up I develop a conversation that I hope will lead to that person either getting a breast check or telling someone they love to get one. It feels comfortable to me and I consider myself skilled enough in the art of conversation to know when to chat about it and when not to.

Surprisingly, many women and some men have cried as I talk through some of the details of my cancer. I have even had nurses cry randomly as they cannulated me or administered medication. Each time I had a new nurse (which was a lot), they would enquire as to how I ended up in the hospital. I would tell them and then they would cry. I didn't cry, but they did, and often. These tears drove my desire to get people talking, in an attempt to remove the social label of breast cancer being a taboo topic and to help others to help themselves. Something was brewing…

Early July 2018 was breast reduction time. For some women, getting a breast reduction is a turning point, even perhaps the highlight of their life. Mine was necessary. This procedure confused people and I often found myself defending this part of my cancer treatment which was chosen for me by the specialists. My plastic surgeon was a perfectionist, which is just what you want when thinking about having your chest reconstructed. The plan was to reduce the size of my left breast – the one that had no cancer – so that when the double mastectomy was carried out, the skin on my breasts would be the same size. As mentioned, the lumpectomy had left my breasts different sizes so this sounded perfectly acceptable to me, but not to others, and I worked hard to not enter into conversation about it as no one seemed to understand. No one wants to have unnecessary surgery, but trusting the surgeons and having faith in what they were offering was all I really had.

The date was set and so was the alarm. Waking up before sunrise was something I did only when I was catching an early flight heading off on holiday, yet here I was on the familiar hospital highway. Registering with the clerk was easy and I got upset only when it was time to weigh myself. I had put on a whopping eight kilos! Thanks, chemo! My mood had changed from very good to feeling disheartened very quickly. Eight kilos. Wasn't having cancer enough of a kick this year?

John's attempts trying to reason with me were futile and I allowed myself to sulk in that moment. It didn't last long, John's perseverance and the fact that I was not going to let my situation dictate my mindset all the time, made me relax a little. It wasn't long before I was taken into the room to check I was who I said I was. More waiting around allowed me to chat with John and crack lots of boob jokes. He was great at keeping the mood light in tense situations. I began pacing up and down, not because I was nervous but to keep warm. One of the nurses provided me with a pair of white compression socks – you know the ones that nobody in the history of ever looks good in? – but they did manage to warm me up. Three anaesthetists came to see me and all said pretty much the same thing, which I thought was strange, but this was not the first time this was to happen.

The third anaesthetist realised I was a bit cold and swiftly brought me a machine called The Bair Hugger System. This really was a game-changer. It's a temperature management system that has a disposable thin blanket placed under the standard blanket and behaves similarly to that of an electric blanket. I was in heat heaven for a while and was miserable when asked to shuffle onto the chilly operating table and my personal sauna was turned off. I always felt lazy when wheeled into theatre and asked to shuffle onto the operating table. Being able-bodied, I was surprised that I wasn't allowed to simply hop off one and onto the other. After the 'octopus' syndrome (many hands doing lots of things to your body at once) was over, I was given the woozy injection, felt the cold mask wrap around my face, a stranger's fingers grip my chin, and a few deep breaths later, it was time for a snooze.

The surgery lasted only three hours. Nerves meant I was hesitant to look at my chest in any capacity for ages. It would take me a further three hours to lift my gown and finally inspect the results. I'm so glad I did! I have to admit, they looked amazing! I stared at them for a long time. They were lovely, curvy, perfectly shaped large C cup-sized breasts and I was beaming. I wasn't alone. John appeared at the bathroom door and couldn't get the smile off his face. 'He really is a perfectionist', he remarked.

After only one night's stay, I was discharged from the hospital and was bringing the now tidy and rather perky twins home. At home, I had to sleep on my back again. The lumpectomy had forced that, so as I was a stomach sleeper by nature, I'd often pine for just one night's reprieve. It would be three weeks before I was able to even side-sleep after the breast reduction, but it didn't matter because I was in love with my new breasts. Nothing could wipe the smile off my face. Little did I know I came home with more than I bargained for, but it was to take five months for anyone to realise this.

Lennox had been emotional. He was a little boy with a lot to deal with. He wanted to sleep with me that night and I caved. In the past, co-sleeping had never been something I had ever done, but our little boy needed me. Besides, it gave me time to study his handsome face. He was a 'hundred miles an hour' type kid, curious about the world around him and had a knack of sweet-talking me! It was lovely going to sleep to the sound of his quiet breathing. Before I slept, I spotted a pile of tissues on his side of my bed. It made me so sad to think they carried the tears of our son.

In the morning after Lennox roused, the first thing he asked was, 'Mum, will you ever get cancer again?' What an incredibly difficult question to answer, and so early!! I had vowed to be truthful to our children, always, but I desperately didn't want to answer him. Words jammed in my throat, but I went with, 'It's a possibility, son' and then skirted over the subject. He had enough to cope with right now, but ultimately, that was our reality. I smiled at the seriousness of his early morning question.

With Layla, I had found surplus 'free time' on my hands. It meant I had time to truly listen to her and talk about anything we felt like. Layla had to mature quickly; she had no choice, but this came pretty easily to her. She was growing up so fast. I could see it right before my eyes. It became hard to look at our children thinking what could have been, but the brain is a machine and knew not to go too deeply with such thoughts. It stopped me from entering a potentially awful state.

Nine

Radiate through radiation

'It felt like such a nice change from chemotherapy at first, but by the end, it was like thinking you had met someone really nice, then you get to know them and they're actually a bitch.'
Sam Thomas – cancer survivor

Late July 2018, my breast surgeon had organised for me to meet with a radiation oncologist at Genesis Care Centre at Frankston Private Hospital to discuss receiving radiation therapy. Martine accompanied me because John was unavailable. I asked permission to record the conversation, allowing John to remain involved without being present – a tip that my support group thought was genius! Perusing the Genesis website not only helped me gain an insight into what I'd be in for over the next months; it also assisted me to find the radiation oncologist's professional photograph – I was really curious as to what he might look like. I pondered for a moment why I was doing this because, if I'm honest, I had done it with my breast surgeon too. I realised I was trying to see who in fact would be responsible for playing a part in saving my life. It makes me laugh when I think of doing it. What was I looking for? I suppose I just wanted to check their skill levels and history. My trust *had* to reside with my breast surgeon as she was the one referring me. May I say, she chose wisely.

It was comforting to have Martine with me. We checked in and didn't wait long before I was sitting in front of the guy responsible for 'mopping up' any remnants of cancer cells in my body. Nerves must've gripped me because, on the transfer from the waiting room to his office, I found myself telling him that I'd recently changed all my underarm deodorants to aluminium-free now, but that I wasn't happy as I felt they didn't last long and blah, blah, blah. I interrupted myself and politely introduced Martine. It was time to find out how he was going to shrink and roast the cells that remained!

Genesis upholds the philosophy of: 'We treat the person, not just the cancer.' I have to say straight off the bat, this is unbelievably true. My radiation oncologist – tall and lean with a pleasant smile – once seated, dropped his chair down to eye level. This felt comforting and I immediately liked him. I signalled to Martine to record the conversation. Now for some unknown reason – possibly chemotherapy haze, tiredness or just being forty-four and not as digitally savvy as I would like – I signalled for Martine to hold down the microphone on an app rather than using the voice recorder and leaving that beside him, hands-free. The meeting ran for around an hour and, every now and again, I could hear Martine shifting in her seat, huffing and puffing and making tiny sounds, as though she were in pain. Each time I glanced across, she would raise her hand and shake her head signalling for me to remain focused.

The oncologists informed me that I would be having what they call EBRT – external beam radiation therapy – something I was familiar with as both Sean and Roisin had been given this type of treatment. Waves of guilt thrashed through my body for the lack of curiosity I showed to them at the time and because I hadn't asked many questions. I rationalised it by thinking I had been more concerned with how they were managing their emotions rather than the ins and outs of how the machinery operated.

I learned that the machine (linear accelerator) uses high energy beams that had one purpose – to destroy cancer cells. I liked the emphasis the oncologist placed on the word 'destroy'. As he said it, it brought me comfort. He further explained that I would have to have 'the big beam', as I nicknamed it, for five weeks, Monday to Friday every day. That was a long time. He said this was to allow time for the healthy cells to repair and the cancer cells to die. I would also receive it to the armpit (axilla) too because of the cancer found there, which made sense.

MARTINE:

'Lindsey asked me to record what the specialist had to say. I focussed so hard on keeping my finger on the record button. After ten minutes cramp set in, but I refused to let go. I recall my finger being sore for days, but, in the scheme of what Lindsey was going through, it was a small price. We still laugh about it now!'

I arrived for my trial run. It began by sitting in with the nurse on-site, where she weighed me and checked me over, giving Genesis a clear idea of my overall health. With so many caregivers and specialists currently looking after me, it was slightly confusing who to ask if anything were to go wrong! I was handed a bright blue, cloth fabric bag with GENESIS on the front. I was provided with an information booklet, which I did read, and was asked to dress in the provided soft blue dressing gown.

I was then taken into the trial run room. This was a space with a table identical to the one I was due to lie on in only a few short days. There were two radiation therapists there and once on the table, my head was then gently lowered onto a firm support. I was instructed to place my arms over my head and into 'arm stirrups' while gripping two small poles. This was to practise which position would be more comfortable for me for the remainder of my radiation sessions. All around me the two therapists buzzed, chatted 'science speak' and made relevant notes about me. They told me the beam had to be very precise when being administered as the healthy tissue around the tumour site had to be protected.

One of my favourite videos of my sister, and there are a few, is the day she celebrated her final radiation session in the U.K. second time around. As a final farewell, she filmed herself in her garden doing the biggest kick of her mesh face mould used to keep her still during radiation all the way down the garden stairs and it hitting the ground. She called it her final farewell. It was done in slow motion and I couldn't help but think how fabulous it looked. She kisses it, lines it up and goes for it. The mould flies through the air, bounces right in line with the camera and comes to rest. She literally kicked it to the kerb!

In the trial run, imaging scans are also taken to establish the precise shape, size and location of the treatment site. They called this the mapping session. To maintain this accuracy, they have to tattoo you. Yes, tattoo, as in forever tattoos – not the ones that wear off over the next few years, even though that would be a good idea, forever! I have two pre-existing tattoos of my own. I had them done following the birth of my children. I have a small red star on the inside of my right wrist for Layla and a small blue star on the outside of the same wrist for Lennox. I'm serious when I say this, but as soon as I had the second tattoo done, wrist tattoos became a trend and were dotted all over social media. Stars, love hearts and names, literally everywhere. I wondered if I had started that trend… Who was I kidding? Get over yourself, Lindsey!

Anyway, I was to have four blue ink dots tattooed on me. The first was respectfully inked dead centre in the middle of my sternum that was still slightly tender following the breast reduction. It was a very different feeling from the buzz of a tattoo needle. It felt more like that feeling you got from stabbing yourself with your compass in maths class because the algebra that your teacher expected you to understand looked and sounded foreign to you! The second and third dots felt equally strange and were placed on my sides, while the fourth one was to the rear of my right underarm. Coming home and telling my children I had four new tattoos meant, for a brief moment in time, I was cool.

Following the tattoos, I was given a timetable of my appointments for the upcoming week. I immediately spotted a 7:30 am appointment and panicked a little. Out of choice I wasn't working, so I was free to do any time, but my children would have to come with me. I explained this to the secretary and she simply smiled and said, 'Bring them. We love children here.' Perfect. I instantly felt better. I was all set. I understood what was going to happen to me over the next five weeks; I had gone through the practice session and knew what my role was in this with regards to body positioning. I just now had to enjoy my weekend and prepare for Monday. Nothing could go wrong, right?

My first session went without incident. I was greeted and directed to get changed and I came out rocking the blue dressing gown like a boss. Soon after, I was ushered into the radiation room and reminded of how big that machine really was. It was absolutely huge and sat alone in a very large room. I asked them for a machine selfie which made them all laugh. I got one with our children and even one of the staff jumped in a photo with me too!

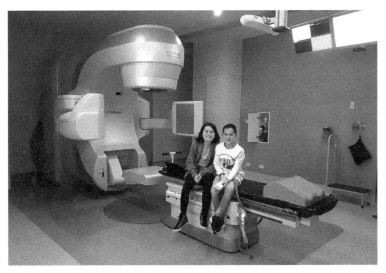

Layla and Lennox perched on the machine with the 'big beam'!

Once placed on the bed, I was respectfully asked to open my dressing gown and they set to work positioning me. It felt strange lying there with my newly shaped breasts exposed to strangers, yet, for the last six months, it had not been an issue. I was told to keep my clothes on from the waist down, which I was grateful for as I was feeling a little self-conscious about the extra kilograms that had set up camp all over my body! They used the dressing gown to move and manipulate me into position and spoke to each other in what appeared to be 'direction and number tongue': 'SUP 5, ANT 4.' The machine had huge moving parts and I came to learn that they were saying the positioning numbers to gain absolute accuracy each time I was zapped.

Seeing my bloated reflection in a mirrored surface left me feeling frustrated about my weight gain. I'd been so fit in January just before diagnosis. Now I was bald and overweight. I quickly reassured myself that it was temporary; I'm good at that. They let me know that they were going to leave the room and be back soon, but if I was uncomfortable in any way, they could hear everything and to just call out. They also made mention of the fact that they would play music for relaxation purposes and dim the lights. Suddenly, I felt so alone. I found my mind wondering about who had lain here before me? How were they now? Did they burn? Did it hurt? Then a timely fun thought crossed my mind: I have a choice – karaoke or meditate?

The staff left, closing the oversized submarine-style door behind them, giving me the most important rule of all, 'Do not move. Be as still as you can.' Then, as promised, they dimmed the main lights revealing twinkle lights on the ceiling. I inhaled deeply and slowly exhaled. A small jolt of the table was a future indication that radiation was about to start. The whir of the robotic machine was LOUD, very loud, but very quick. I couldn't believe it. In my head, I just thought it would be long and hot, like roasting a chicken.

Neither karaoke nor meditation happened because it was so quick. The machine rotated from my front to my side several times and I could see a red dot – the big beam that radiated me. During that session, I imagined the cancer cells exploding and dying as the moving mirrored plates looked like large T-Rex-style teeth, and it brought me instant relief. Treatment was painless and not what I had expected. I imagined it to be like x-ray eyes that cut around steel doors in superhero movies.

Session one was now over. One down, twenty-four to go. Moisturiser was provided in the change rooms post-radiation, which was very important to me, and I had no qualms soaking the radiated area with the stuff. I had also been discouraged from shaving under my armpit and using deodorant to reduce the risk of any damage to the skin in the radiated area.

The second session made me miserable and I still don't know why. I quietly cried, which was a bad idea as my crying was discovered because it was over so quickly. I decided with all further treatments I would embrace them, think positively and allow myself to be in the moment while under the control of 'the big beam.'

I began to wear lavender oil to relax before my sessions at this point. I took Layla and Lennox to the third session, due to circumstance. The children coming to radiation with me helped them to demystify what I was going through. They saw first-hand just how well taken care of Mummy was. They also loved the fact that there were free mints at the front desk and developed a habit of having one on arrival and then reminding me how well-behaved they'd been to earn another as we left! The staff really did love children, and they treated Layla and Lennox like gold. My children have never struggled in any public arena. I'm always proud of the way they conduct themselves. Okay, being honest, I may have once become a little stressed when it was footy day at Genesis and Lennox ate his body weight in party pies and sausage rolls! Over time, the staff built up a beautiful rapport with our children.

Another extraordinary thing that took place during my connection to Genesis was the relationship Layla formed with the manager, Luke, and two of his staff. She struck up a conversation with Luke because he had a fifty-centimetre, bright green alien peering out of his office window that drew her attention. She quizzed him about it and he suggested Layla might want to take it home and look after it for the weekend. She was holding a cuddly, soft, toy dog named Pablo with huge eyes which she quickly asked to trade. He graciously accepted.

She named the alien Luke Skywalker on the spot and over the next few days, it went everywhere with her. It reminded me of when she was in Grade One at school and had to look after a fluffy toy wombat and keep a diary of the wombat's adventures. I loved the way this stimulated her imagination. So many photos of Layla and Luke Skywalker were taken which she went on to happily display for her friends in the classroom scrapbook. Luke and Layla eventually swapped back and shared stories and photos of the adventures taken. At the end of my radiation, Layla and Luke did something wonderful. They exchanged gifts. Luke got to keep Pablo and Layla got to keep Luke Skywalker.

Two other friendships born were with Happy and Dianne, who was known as Di. Layla had no qualms in letting Di know that her name was rather inappropriate given that radiation therapy was supposed to help save your life! She agreed. Happy was just amazing and lived up to her name. She is literally the happiest person we know. The three of them became great mates and Layla lit up when she came to Genesis with me.

I was very pleased there was no redness of my skin or a feeling of burning. I had hoped that I'd be one of the lucky ones who simply escaped radiation reactions. Eventually, I did end up with a slightly pink breast and armpit and I attest this to the amount of moisturiser I used. I had started wearing crop tops for support rather than no underwire bras as the rubbing can aggravate the skin.

It was after the fourth session that I noticed the breast reduction scar on my right breast was slightly oozing and turning red and green. Red I could understand, but green got me worried. When I arrived home and checked in the mirror, my front-zipped bra was wet on the right side. This was one of those confusing moments. Do I call the breast surgeon as it is in the breast area? Do I call the cosmetic surgeon because he did the surgery? Do I call my radiation oncologist because I am currently in his care? Do I go to the hospital because it doesn't look or feel right?

I decided to call Genesis to speak to a nurse and get some advice. She advised me to come straight back. When I arrived, my radiation oncologist confirmed that I had an infection and that I'd have to go on a course of antibiotics and cease treatment immediately. I was to have a two-week break from radiation. I was deflated and disappointed but knew it was just par for the course. It was July 30th and this 'situation' turned out to be unbelievably problematic, to say the least.

During my treatment, some days I was more tired than others, but I don't think that at any time I was overwhelmed by tiredness. It was accumulative, and when I felt fatigued, I would just have a nanna nap. Radiation can be a little taxing emotionally because you have to go there every day, but I was strong like an ox, strong mentally. During my two-week break from

Genesis, I made what I consider a fabulous decision. I needed to start filling my days with positive activities, as I knew that being still or bored did not work for me.

I enrolled in a course. Early August saw me break out of the safety net of teaching and look at another career path. People did it all the time, didn't they? I once met a teacher in his forties who was on his fifth career choice. Back then, I thought that was really brave. I registered for my Certificate IV in Civil Celebrancy. On the application form, it asked why I wanted to become a civil celebrant. I wrote:

> '*Earlier this year, I was diagnosed with an illness that made me reassess what happiness really is. I was in a job that I loved, but I knew that I wasn't being as fulfilled as what I could be in my life. I have always worked with people and wanted to keep that the same. I am a naturally vibrant person with a genuine zest for life.*
>
> *Five years ago, I attended a wedding in country Victoria where I fell in love with the celebrant, not the actual celebrant, just his capacity to unite my two friends so beautifully on their special day. I left that wedding thinking about celebrancy and how it was a potential path for me. I was excited, knowing that I had the potential to have a future filled with love and positivity.*
>
> *I love people, I love love and I love a chat.*'

I was in! I interviewed well and began the course. It was more intense than I expected, with several fairly lengthy assignments and many oral presentations. I got to work immediately, and on and off spent around eight hours on assignment one.

Now, somewhere in between my house and the printers, the unbelievable happened. I LOST the USB that had assignment one on it and had not backed it up on my laptop. I was distraught. I slammed down hard on my desk, hurting my hands and scaring the dog! This event then saw me have a huge meltdown. I had never experienced anything like it. I was feeling emotions I'd never felt before and realised that all my stress since late January had accumulated. Today was the day I was releasing that pressure. I cried for bloody ages. I gave up after four hours of searching and looked at myself in the mirror for a long time. What had happened to me? I was in despair and was talking out loud to myself at this point. 'What were you thinking, Lindsey? You can't do a course – chemotherapy has stripped you of your senses! You have stumbled at the first hurdle! Just stick to what you know!'

I rang John after a little sleep, knowing that I was calm enough. I talked it through with him and found reason. The next day I got up and reluctantly started on assignment one again. Just to kick me while I was down, using a computer more made me realise that my eyesight was a little blurry. Off I went to the opticians and three weeks later found myself reliant on glasses for reading. Was this a side effect of treatment or my age? I guess I'll never really know.

Life carried on and I soon began getting into a smooth radiation routine. Even though I had to re-start my five weeks of therapy from scratch because of the infection, this time there were no further problems… yet! In the end, I had completed twenty-nine treatments over seven weeks and I managed just fine.

When friends asked me what it felt like, I told them, 'It was nothing. I felt nothing.' I rewarded myself with some retail therapy with the children. As I shopped, a lady spotted my headscarf and said, 'Ahhhhh, do you have cancer?' WOW! I let her know that it was a thing of the past and I was just having radiation at the moment. It wasn't a long conversation before we smiled and parted ways. Outside, Layla told me that she nearly responded with, 'Ahhhhh, do you have manners?' It made me laugh. Her protective instinct had kicked in and I explained that the lady was just making an observation. She didn't agree. 'No, Mum. It's just rude.' I could see where she was coming from as John also let me know that the headscarves I wore always got looks. He seemed to notice the things I didn't. He saw those sideways glances somewhat laden with pity. At the mall, people do stare. Why is that? Curiosity, I hoped.

On the radiation 'home straight', I received two phone calls two days apart that threw me. Two of my close friends were diagnosed with early-stage breast cancer. I was angry – really angry – and became more intent on creating something which would get people sitting up and listening. I started to put a little bit of time and energy into an initiative that I could present in thirty minutes. It needed more work, but I knew I was onto something.

At the same that I was undergoing radiation, my sister was doing the same in the U.K. Our lives were running parallel again and it felt good to be so close. I missed her so much and was pained when I thought of what she was going through. On my last day, John had a sneaky surprise in store for me. He'd organised some friends to be at Genesis when I arrived for my final radiation. What a sweetheart! I was elated. It was a perfect reflection of how my journey had been so far. Being consistently loved, nurtured and cared for by these wonderful people left me feeling genuinely valued.

I prepared myself for the final hot blast. As I walked into the radiation room, Happy had been on a love mission, covering the walls with posters of rainbows and sunflowers. They were everywhere. There was an unspoken connection to Roisin and I had an extra spring in my step.

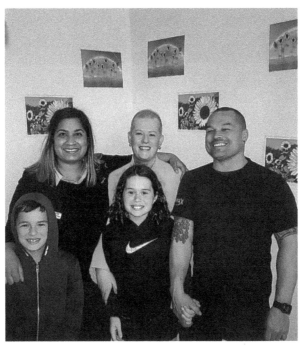

Happy, myself, John and the children all smiles
as we knew this would be my last radiation therapy.

Suddenly I heard my dad's voice, then my mum's, my four brothers and my superstar sister through the speakers. They were leaving very personal love messages to me and lots of encouraging well wishes. This was unreal! I just loved that my romantic husband had contacted all my immediate family in the U.K. asking them to send a message to me. The staff members were even in on it. I was bawling under that machine, absolutely bawling.

Walking away from this journey with so many people around me was great, but the physical distance between me and my family was poignant in this moment and I allowed myself to wish they were here. When the robotic arm finally fell silent, successful in its quest, I thanked it, said goodbye to it and told it in the nicest possible way that I would never like to see it ever again (insert profanity here).

Radiation had just been one part of the bigger puzzle that was going to put me back together again.

Ten

'There's something I need to get off my chest.'

'I'll miss those cushions.'
Lennox Kennedy

It was the right decision that just went wrong.
Feeling excited but scared to death is a weird paradigm for anyone to be in.

I had decided early on that my breasts had to go – drastic to some, but necessary to me. I knew from the moment of Roisin's first diagnosis that, if I would ever be unfortunate enough to be diagnosed with breast cancer, then a double mastectomy would be the best course of action for me. It would only be a short five years later that I'd have to make this awful decision for myself. Revealing this publicly meant that the odd person would, unfortunately, sit in judgement of my skin and nipple-sparing surgery decision (for the eventual reconstruction) saying such things as, 'I don't know why you would put yourself through all that pain. They're just boobs, you've had your babies and they've done their job', or 'Get rid of them, I would.' They asked why I would put myself through that when there is no sign of cancer after my lumpectomy.

This forced me to think people should be careful with their words. Ultimately, these were the decisions that I made for *myself* about *my* health. I saw a mastectomy as a solution, as the best-case scenario for *me*. I was only forty-four years old and I didn't want to be flat-chested for the rest of my life! Of course, there were going to be times when I would miss my ex-baby feeders and even though they were big and rather saggy, they were okay. I had to just shrug those statements off and sit comfortably with *my* decision. I deserved this choice. I may have been forty-four on the outside, but my spirit was still twenty-four. Feeling like others were being a bit judgemental about my personal decision didn't affect me too much. I was raised to be resilient – to have thick skin. I just took it as people misunderstanding my choice and that, of course, is fine.

People would also refer to my experience as having a 'tummy tuck' and 'boob job'. I believe such statements trivialised what I had to go through. 'Yeah people, I only had to get cancer to look like this!' 'I'll give you some of my fat' was a comment also tossed around by many. A moot point but kudos for trying to throw light on the subject! The decision to remove my breasts was not for vanity or appearance's sake; rather, I elected to replace body parts that had tried to kill me.

Images of our beautiful children regularly had floated past my eyes and it was easy after that. I didn't want the internal bashing I would give myself if I only removed one and it came back in the other breast later on. That was it, decision made, even without genetic testing. For me, it was a no-brainer!

One day, I was with our children at the clinic having my blood taken by a rather jovial young nurse. She was asking how I was and went on to tell us of her own sister's battle with breast cancer. The details of the story were not heading in the direction of survival and she slowly mouthed to me, so the children could not tell what she was saying, 'She died'. I couldn't believe it. Our children may not have seen it, but lady, I did! Fun tip #1: Don't tell a person diagnosed with breast cancer that you know of someone who's died of breast cancer. Being on the receiving end of such comments has made me realise the negative powers behind such fleeting statements.

Thoughtless and flippant comments about any topic can hurt and now I am far more mindful when I speak to others about sensitive issues, not just cancer. If you need to comment on a person's situation, please do so with empathy and sensitivity. I will now conclude my whinge with the worst cancer statement of all time: 'A whole new upper body! What more could you ask for? Lucky you!' LUCKY! I think not. It's traumatic. THINK before you speak, people. It's a mastectomy, not a makeover!

Leaving the cosmetic surgeon's office earlier in the year had left me with the understanding that the procedure called a DIEP would be using my lower abdomen skin and abdominal fat (autologous) and transferring it to my chest to make a breast that would produce a soft, warm, natural look and feel. Skin sparing – keeping my own breast skin – and nipple-sparing – keeping my nipples – would also be part of my plan. I had left that day comfortable I'd been referred to a plastic surgeon in the upper echelon of surgeons. There were criteria I had to satisfy: I had to be reasonably fit, which I was, and I had to have healthy blood vessels in my abdomen. I also had to have enough fat to form my original breast size, even though going smaller was highly probable. This was something I was more than comfortable with.

Had I been preparing for this in the past? I amused myself thinking that I had secretly been storing stomach fat in preparation for this operation. At home and standing in front of my full-length mirror (yes, I own a full-length mirror – haters, don't hate) found me squishing my stomach and attempting to mould it into a breast shape. I'm currently sitting crimson-red-faced, remembering that I did this (or it could be a hot flush?). I begged myself to stop doing it because it was weird, but I couldn't and it made me hysterical with laughter.

I started to learn more about this mammoth operation. I needed 'layman's terms'. Two almond-shaped sections of skin, tissue and blood vessels were to be taken from my stomach and placed into my chest cavity. Once transferred, the tissue would be joined up to blood vessels underneath the ribs using a microscope to restore blood flow to the tissue. This was to be some decent 21st century plumbing. My body would then be very carefully stitched back together. I imagined hearing chants of 'Heave' as many hands would work in unison to close me. The icing on the cake was when purple glue would ensure I didn't come undone.

Preparation for my life-altering surgery was in full swing. It began with my friend, 'Kim Boobs', as she has endearingly become known (also a DIEP recipient). She is a massage therapist by trade and I was so blessed to have her work on my body for many hours to prepare me for its weeks of stillness. I would make Layla and Lennox laugh by practising getting on and off the toilet seat, in fact, any seat, without using my arms. Every little building block I put in place pre-op was to make life run smoothly post-op.

Two days before my surgery my friend, Renee, organised a 'bye-bye booby' afternoon tea complete with the most brilliant set of boobs in a lacy bra cake made by Mel. I loved it and I loved them for throwing humour on my serious medical decision.

Before surgery, I had to have a CT scan of my lower abdomen. The intravenous contrast dye used wasn't painful but did give me the sensation of wetting my pants, but I pinky-promise you, I didn't.

Surgery, now referred to as D-Day (DIEP Day), was booked for the day after Lennox's ninth birthday, October 15th. Doubt crept in as the date drew near, then went away, crept in and went away like the quiet ebb and flow of an ocean wave. My mind went into overdrive and questions fired in quick succession. Was I being selfish? I mean, the surgery had such a long recovery, our children were young and still needed me. Had I made the right decision to remove both breasts instead of just the cancer side? Who was I keeping my breasts for – me or us? Should I just elect to remove them completely, skin and all? Was I going to feel mutilated after the fact? Then, the big one – what if I died on the operating table? It happens. Trust me when I say, this was an awful predicament to be in. I had never been selfish in life, ever. I believe in life there are givers and takers and I was a definite giver. So many thoughts and questions prefaced my sleep and this went on for some time.

Right before my surgery, I received awful news. A few months earlier, my McGrath Foundation contact, who just had a knack of knowing what I needed, had connected me with a lady called Julie whom I was only ever to text, but never to meet. We had exchanged chatter over multiple weeks and found out that we'd undergone similar diagnoses and treatments. I could tell through her texts that I would like her, that she was my kind of lady – funny, strong, energetic and brave. We had attempted to arrange to meet multiple times over a few months but to no avail. Every time she happened to be free, I wasn't and vice versa.

Finally, the day came for us to meet. With our children packed off to school, we decided that I would go to her place and we would talk the morning away. We planned for ten o'clock as she had a doctor's appointment. With a worried tone in her voice, she called me to say I had to stay away as she had developed shingles. I had never had shingles but I knew that with my immune system compromised at the moment, her place had to be a no-go zone. Yet again, we had failed to meet.

Not too long after this, I read online that Julie had gone to have her annual check-up and that her cancer was back. I was devastated for her. She'd been given a terminal diagnosis. The cancer had spread through her body like a snowstorm and she was looking at less than six months to live. I burst into tears immediately and my heart broke for someone I didn't even know. For the first time in ten months, reality smacked me in the face.

I write often that I am positive, have a strong mindset and constantly remind myself that life is going to be great, but not this day. My family was home so I avoided them and hopped in the shower for a cry, sobbing as quietly as I could. My tears were multi-layered. I cried for my new acquaintance as I was desperately sad for her, I cried for the friendship that I never got to have, and I cried because I was so utterly scared to death about a recurrence for me. It was the first time that I'd thought about the reality of my cancer coming back. I thought long and hard about how both my grandmothers had battled cancer twice, how my sister had battled cancer twice and how Sean had endured cancer twice. There was a pattern there, a theme. Was I looking at life through rose-coloured glasses again, thinking that there were no flies on me? I owned the attitude of '*I live in the lucky country. She'll be right*'. Was I being completely naïve and should I be more concerned?

I cried for so long over the next few days. Julie was so young and she had already battled with cancer, but most of all I cried because this terrible disease killed her and took her away from all that she knows. My mortality was in question and I knew it. I had to work hard mentally to recover from this. The news of this terminal diagnosis rocked me to say the least. I wobbled and it made things very real for me.

Another blow in the 'year that was' came five days before D-Day. A friend of mine, Jessie, died of a brain tumour. Life is God-damned cruel sometimes. She was far too young to die. She was one of life's greats and most certainly had not finished at 'life' yet. She hadn't finished being a wife, a friend, a daughter, and most of all she had not finished being a mum. She taught me to love every minute of my life, no matter how many minutes I had left. I learned to adore 'the little things' in my life on a deeper level because of Jess. Now, when I watch our children sleep, I absorb all that they are, and I pause to appreciate them. During my treatments, Jessie had called *me* to check in on *me* when she was so unbelievably ill – an act that is a real testament to her character and something that I will never forget.

Martine and Cindy had organised for all our families to go out for dinner the night before my surgery. In the restaurant, observing all the smiles, banter and interactions of my family and friends, helped me feel super-relaxed. We left our children with Martine's family that night to take over the routine of bedtime and school, and John had booked a hotel room in the city, close to the hospital.

When we arrived at the rather swanky hotel, the front desk clerk enquired as to the purpose of our stay. When we explained, he clutched his chest horrified and stared at my very new duckling style fluffy tufts that were beginning to pop all over my head. He was speechless and remained typing with one hand while his other remained clutched to his chest. He was muttering like a madman to the keyboard on his computer in worried tones, 'No, no, no' and 'Oh no' being the main phrases used.

To our surprise, he asked us to follow him where he escorted us to the penthouse of one of Melbourne's top hotels. It was magnificently grandiose. Things like that just didn't happen to us and we were left excitedly stunned. I had never been in an apartment so big… correction, I had never been in a penthouse apartment full stop! Needless to say, the night before the biggest surgery of my life was nearly perfect. However, the fear of the unknown still ran cold through my veins. I just hoped that this fear would be greater than the pain I was about to endure. Viewing my surgery as simply getting rid of something that had the potential to cause future problems kept me on the right side of sane.

In the morning, John and I made our way to the admission unit where they routinely confirmed my details. It didn't take long to be weighed, my blood pressure taken and allergy information recorded. Interestingly, on this occasion, I was asked to recite the alphabet backwards. Swift success left the nurse astonished. She was amazed at how flawless and quick I was. I felt happy with my efforts back then, but I tried to do this recently and it was a complete disaster with a speed similar to that of a five year-old child. Realistically, there has been pharmaceutical intervention between the first time and the most recent. At least, that's my excuse!

A preoperative requirement with most surgeries is to be drawn on with blue and black sharpies (skin marking pens). I felt a sudden urge to grab the pen and draw 'Adios' across my chest, but thought better of it. There I stood, my gown fully open, naked in a small room with my surgeon. I had to control my breathing a little because I was so anxious, not about the surgery, but about being so exposed – pardon the pun. In the past I had managed this, but that day it was humiliating.

Following this, a team of doctors and nurses came in to familiarise themselves with the sharpie lines before the surgery. It was super daunting now that I was lying completely naked while they chatted above my body with no one looking me in the eyes. One of the surgeons was using a medical measuring tape for some of the lines and I could see John over his shoulder being ever-so-subtle, but making motions with his hands, mouthing 'massive'. It made me laugh as I shook my head, wide-eyed.

I was my surgeon's first surgery of the day because I was his only surgery of the day and most probably one of the longest surgeries. The next team to greet me was the anaesthetics team. One of them was strikingly tall, very methodical and left us both feeling very comfortable about what was to happen to me during the day. It became John's time to leave. I found this part difficult. Once again, I was petrified of dying on the operating table. I didn't cry but I wanted to.

In theatre, what felt like a shoal of piranhas set upon my body. The nurses commented on how incredibly calm I was and told me I was going to be asleep for a long, long time and to enjoy the rest. I did feel calm at this point. I didn't feel jittery, nervous or anxious anymore. I felt strong. I guess I'd had enough time to think about my choice to remove my breasts and I had dwelt on it enough.

Once again, I had to place myself in the hands of the medical staff. I thought of the procedure one final time and winced when I imagined the breast surgeon scraping out my natural breast tissue from my chest and armpits with a great big ice-cream scoop while I was asleep. I have no idea how it was done and really don't care to know. It's scary to think that I was going through all this and that cancer, in fact, might never return. But by having a prophylactic mastectomy, I knew I was doing everything possible to stop cancer revisiting my body. I took a deep breath, and just like the lumpectomy, I thought, 'There's no going back now'. The strength to get through this was inside me and I slowly thought of Layla's, Lennox's and John's faces.

The piranha effect slowed, multiple instructions stopped, a mask was placed on my face and there was only the smoke alarm left to stare at. After a few more deep breaths and a last thought of, 'Oh good God, they're all going to see my vagina', they pushed the sleepy drugs and I was gone. Unbeknown to my medical team, mayhem was about to be unleashed upon my body.

Twelve hours and fifty minutes later felt as though I had just blinked. I heard a stranger's voice calling my name over and over. I woke up thinking about how wonderful it felt to have survived such a big procedure. I tried to ask what time it was, but I had no energy to move my lips. Placed in the high dependency unit, I saw a familiar red t-shirt. Acknowledging John was there with the smallest of smiles, I immediately fell back to sleep. I had made it.

In the hospital, I got to know the nurses very well. Over time, and when dealing with a plethora of health professionals, I only ever had one bad nurse experience. I consider that really good odds. Anyone who played a part in my care was just lovely, kind, warm and understanding. Then there was one nurse…

My friend, Shelley, had accompanied me to a hospital appointment one day and the nurse responsible for taking my blood was angry from the get-go. She struggled to read the handwriting of one of my care team and was whinging about it. This whinge became more intense and, before we knew it, 'Nurse Ratchet' (from *One Flew Over the Cuckoo's Nest*) was full-on raging about how she was expected to do her job when a doctor could not grasp the basics of cursive script. I darted my eyes in the direction of Shelley to see her eyes large and round. I knew I couldn't look at Shelley again for fear I would burst into laughter. Then, Nurse Ratchet swore. Before I knew it, I was lecturing her. I very calmly told her she was too angry and aggressive for me and to go and get someone else. She hastily left the room, still grumpy. She returned with a lady whom I recognised. Nurse Ratchet popped her head back in over the shoulder of my new nurse remarking, 'This lady thinks that I can't do my job and she wants me replaced.' I did not satisfy her with an answer. I just nodded.

The new nurse managed the situation and, with that, Grumpy was gone. I explained that sometimes what was going on in our own lives can be projected onto others and that I had only become cross when she swore in front of me and my friend. Leaving the room, Shelley and I turned into two giggling schoolgirls. It reminded me of being at school when you are not allowed to laugh so you hold your breath or your nose. It was a small but strange victory.

During my hospital stay following my mastectomy, a lady popped in to show me how to breathe properly following such a big operation. I was too afraid to take a great big breath because I felt like if I did, I would be in excruciating pain. I was shallow breathing quite often to play it safe. I was encouraged to take five deep breaths every hour, otherwise I could be prone to lung infections, and this was to be finished off with a cough. A cough? I tried to keep my face as straight as possible when she told me this but what I wanted to shout was, 'Are you kidding me?' Coughing proved near impossible and day three saw me manage the most pitiful sounding cough. It makes me grin remembering how pathetic it sounded. As for sneezing, well that's a different matter entirely! I was dreading the aftershock.

Early the next day, I noticed that there was a yellow stain on my pillow in the divot where my head had been. The nurse inspected the back of my head where she could see a very small, pimple-sized blister. It seemed to be nothing to worry about, especially in relation to other things I was enduring. My stomach had been pulled closed and my belly button had to be relocated. The surgeon had cut around the belly button and left it there, then pulled it through a new hole after the upper abdomen skin has been pulled down. Freaky, right? My new belly button is nicer than the old one, even though Lennox says it resembles a cat's bottom!

Due to my incapacitation, oversized hospital body wipes were used to bed-bath me and I felt like a giant baby! It was impossible to shower and, as it turns out, this was to be the case for the next seventy-seven days! Right from the beginning, my breasts were a funny colour – a green-yellowy-reddish blue. They looked like they were not behaving themselves and the doctors were worried.

There is nothing glamorous about the next paragraph, feel free to skip it. I won't be offended. I nearly named this book *The Nitty-Gritty* because I discuss many areas in and around what has happened to me in detail, sort of a behind-the-scenes look at a breast cancer diagnosis. One area of self-care that's very difficult to speak about… hold on, breathe… just let me find my bravery badge… is… toileting. There, I said it. Post DIEP, I could not wipe my own bottom as my shoulders, waist and arms weren't working that well. Phew, that was hard. I simply could not manage.

So, how did I do it when my arms were temporarily unavailable? This was the lowest point in my life, EVER, no exaggeration. I chose the nurses to assist with the job at hand instead of my husband as, even though I felt shy, they were very experienced with that kind of thing. Even though John and I had said 'in sickness and in health' in our wedding vows, I felt this particular job had the potential to do permanent damage to John's eyeballs!

The nurses were so supportive. They put me on a commode. This would assist me using the toilet for the next few days. The nurses would come into the toilet when I rang the bell, fix me up and chat happily all the while. In the meantime, I was reduced to silence, which is so very rare for me. To be honest, I was mortified; it was mortifying. I willed myself to overcome all the pain and I tried to force myself to reach but to no avail. It was so tough and some of the hardest days of my life. I cried and cried after the first time, but because of my bloody shoulder restriction, I couldn't even wipe my tears away. It was just too painful! This was not glamorous at all. How could I relax when another fully grown adult was doing that to me? I spent a lot of time in the bathroom waiting for my bowels to play nice because of the medications I was on and, quite often, it took a while before my body decided to obey. Eventually, I was able to reach but it took me a good while. Enough of that now; it's torture reliving those moments!

A week later and it was time to get my drains removed. I had four altogether – one at the bottom of each breast and one in each side/flank area. Their job was to drain blood slowly away from my incisions. I was a little nervous about the removal but I shouldn't have been as it was very manageable. Taking a deep breath in, the nurse pulled out the drains on my exhale. I was flabbergasted to see how long they were, on average around twenty-five centimetres!

Layla and Lennox came to see me only once during that week. I may have had other visitors but it was all a bit of a blur. John's priority was our children, and with the hospital being over an hour away and us wanting to keep up their usual routines of school and sports, I entertained myself most days. When I did see Layla, she once told me she had dreamt she was swimming with a feeling that she was looking for something. I asked what was she was looking for and she replied, 'I think it was your health, Mum.' I choked back tears and heard my heart break a little. Reaching across the bed, I held her hand, reassuring her once again that I had this.

At this point, I'm hurting. I'm hurting emotionally, but also physically. I wanted to cry but I knew it hurt to cry, so thought better of it. John attempted to make me laugh; he was good at that. I had to ban him from talking to me at times because my supersized stomach scar did not appreciate his sense of humour. John is a happy, smiley and hilarious character and someone whose company people enjoy. I was miserable when my family left at night and found myself questioning every decision I had made in this whole situation. To make matters worse, this was the day of the sneeze! The sneeze was hell and left me filled with dread for the next one.

A physiotherapist came to do a review in preparation for me going home. Dressed in a front-zipped hoodie, my thoughts turned to counselling. I thought standard policy should be to offer all mastectomy patients mental health support before leaving to go home because, in my case, let's face it, I had been surgically sawn in half and my stomach was used to create two new lady lumps. All this led to one daunting thought. Someone, at some stage, was going to have to help me put my knickers on!

Once in the car, which was a long slow process in itself, I wanted to blast the song *I'm a Survivor* in the car down St Kilda Rd, but to be honest, there was something wrong. I could feel it in my heart, but I couldn't explain what it was.

I was looking forward to some home creature comforts, hanging out with Layla and Lennox, stroking Melfi and of course, sleeping without any beeping. Sleeping on my stomach has always been my bedroom staple, but because of my enormous incision I was advised to sleep upright again for around six weeks, so the chemo chair and I reunited. Propped up with pillows in numerous places, I was finally home and comfortable. Sleeping on my back was to last months and months. I truly felt like Tutankhamun or a vampire in the end. I came out of my DIEP surgery thinking that was the end of my treatment but, unfortunately, it wasn't the end of my battle.

The end of October 2018 saw the arrival of my parents. I was desperate to pick them up from the airport, but my body had other ideas and held me to ransom in my home. Asking for help from my parents was difficult. It was foreign to me and not something I practised very often. As the eldest daughter in a family of six children, I was always the helper. I had to alter my mindset and move away from the self-reliant me and move towards being someone who had no shame in asking for assistance. Being incapacitated from the hips up left me no choice. The physical distance between my family in the U.K. and us in Melbourne was hard, but we tried to never convert this into emotional distance.

Mum and Dad had not even been on Australian soil for twenty-four hours and we had them working their fingers to the bone! During the first few days, every time I looked at my parents, they were looking at me with 'those eyes'. You know the ones, those eyes that show heartbreak, concern and helplessness. They wanted to take all this away from me, I could feel it. Meanwhile, there was something wrong and I knew it was serious. My left breast was rapidly changing colour. Instead of playing Aussie tourists, they stepped up and took over the running of the house, maintaining everything and keeping Layla and Lennox both occupied and happy, in order for John to return to work as the only breadwinner. The only thing I had to complain about were the hospital car parking fees. It didn't bother me really. As a public patient, that hospital had helped to save my life.

It was time for me to try and resume some normal activities. Shortly after returning home, Layla had her interview to enter high school. I was determined to support her, no matter what. I was three weeks out from my surgery, using a walking stick and still folded in half. Visions of me mimicking the scene in *Willy Wonka and the Chocolate Factory* movie made me beam. Gene Wilder exits the factory slowly with a limp and, as he is face to face with the winning children, he heroically throws himself into a forward roll. There was to be no forward roll for me, however I was about to deal with my own movie – a horror movie!

I made my way to Melbourne city to attend a 'Think Pink' birthday cele-bration. They were turning eight and I felt happy to go, drink tea and mingle. Think Pink is a foundation that provides professional and caring, holistic support completely free of charge to patients, their families and carers at any stage of their journey with breast cancer. It was a lovely afternoon. I always got a sense of family there and remain amazed at how present they were and how good their memories were when I visited. It could be a two- or three-month gap and they'd still remember me and details of my journey.

I chin-wagged with a small group of volunteers, listening intently to their journeys all laden with sadness, terror and of course survival, and I began to note similarities. When it came to me recounting my journey, I could read their faces and in them I saw shock. They were not doing this on purpose, but they were moving their faces in such a way it could only make me realise it was startlingly obvious. Should I have been more worried? I reassured them that cancer was not going to ever get me again or anyone else in my family and they chorused that my sense of optimism should never leave me.

As time passed, my breasts remained all colours of the rainbow. I had developed a small, but obvious pink dot, which was the size of a pea on my right breast. It sat on the nipple scar line from the lumpectomy and over time it started to turn from pink to red. Then it changed from red to purple quite quickly. Again, a few suggestions of what it might be were tossed around, but no one really knew what it was. Over the next few days and now presenting as a deep purple dot, layers of skin would peel off, similar to sunburn. The skin over the ominous dot soon became so thin I could see a thickened, puss-like fluid underneath it, leaving me filled with dread about what might happen if it burst.

The hospital had given me dressings in case the inevitable happened, so I was prepared. I didn't have to wait long. While brushing my teeth before bed that night, I noticed a big orange stain on my top in the bathroom mirror. I quickly checked and there was a hole – literally a hole in my breast and it looked deep. The fluid leaking started off orange then turned slightly green. After the small waterfall in my breast had slowed, I dressed the wound, went to bed and knew to ring the breast clinic first thing in the morning. They requested I see them that very day to take a look at what was going on.

Once there, it was thought to be a stitch abscess due to its position. The best course of action was to have the wound packed. This was very gross and I was happy to not watch. Gauze was dipped in saline and an oversized ear cleaner (jumbo swab stick) was used to track how deep it was. My breasts were still numb at this point, so it wasn't too painful. The hole was then packed as the wound had to heal from the inside out. This whole dramatic event was unfortunately to be the first of many and my life was to become a waiting game, requiring lots and lots of patience.

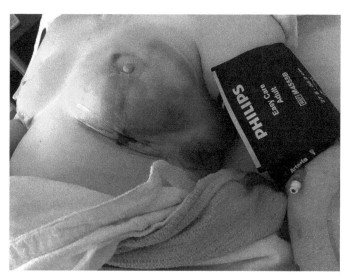

My situation remained a mystery to the doctors for some time.
My left breast rapidly showed signs of ill health.

My breast surgeon encouraged me to join a support group at The Bays Hospital in Mornington. Yes, I had heaps of friends and lots of family, but I needed a support group filled with like-minded women who knew exactly what I was going through. For me, I believed that talking to women who'd experienced breast cancer first-hand gave me great insight, and any advice from others in a like-minded situation was most welcome.

Run by legendary well-loved and well known McGrath Foundation Breast Care Nurses, Jo and Felicity, the monthly gatherings at the hospital offer reassurance, support and care. I have lost count how many times I've used their expertise to help me problem-solve. I love their name too: 'Breast Intentions'. You can't beat it! I have made new friends through this group and love our supportive banter. Before appointments, writing down questions and concerns about my journey, and bringing them up in conversation with my support group has been an enormous help. It sounds mean to say, but friends and family can only understand to a point. Women who have walked a mile in my shoes were great at appeasing me in my times of need.

I was asked recently if I'd recommend the DIEP procedure that I had to someone else. Wow! Such a loaded question caught me off guard. DIEP has had such repercussions on my life for so long I would be inclined to say no, but I went with offering that each woman is different and individual and that it is solely up to them. What I would suggest doing is asking many, many, many questions, doing a risk analysis with your doctors, and getting second and third opinions as part of your own research.

The next step in my cancer treatment was for me to be placed on a drug called tamoxifen. It had one objective: to block the production of estrogen. Estrogen was one of my cancer's food sources and it had to be gone. Tamoxifen couldn't guarantee me that cancer would never return, but I felt better taking it. It became a feeling of self-protection of the highest order. The alternative did not bear thinking about.

Emotionally, it was crazy how quickly things changed. I became teary on tamoxifen, evident when getting dressed one day, I caught myself crying like a Karen Carpenter family member over one of her songs – a memory that I laugh about now. I was unreasonably sad that she had died at thirty-two and that she'd suffered from an eating disorder. I would also cry at advertisements or if someone shared a story that even had a hint of sad news in it. I experienced feelings of 'lost control' and frustratingly, at times, it would get the better of me.

Cognitive change certainly happened and I loved the way Layla and Lennox would step in and act as my memory. I just needed to look at them and they would know I was confused or couldn't get a word out. Charades was to become the number one game in our house. We were forced to invest in an oversized calendar that hopefully would not allow for error, lateness or missed events. That's not to say it didn't happen! I became slightly concerned about my mental capacity and I was losing little grey brain cells on a daily basis.

Hot flushes are so impolite and extremely unpredictable. I was also to endure my first toe-curling hot flush. Blimey! I wanted to leap out of my own body, out of the internal fire. After talking to my doctors, I now know that there is estrogen in many parts of the body. It's around the brain, in the stomach lining, in the heart, in fat cells and the adrenal glands. Estrogen is a great lubricator of the vagina, joints, skin and brain. Entering the phase of menopause had, once again, forced ignorance to rear its ugly head. I just thought menopause was where you had hot flushes because you were changing from a woman to an old-age pensioner… gulp! There was so much more than that. Jo informed me that menopause can last up to fifteen years in some women. Fifteen years! Good Lord, what a community joke! One bloody tumour causing all this disharmony in my body! I allowed myself to be angry and once again and felt completely pissed off.

I spent time thinking about the anatomy of a hot flush. A lady in my support group described her hot flush as '*an ugly feeling coming over her*' and I thought – *that's it*! It really is an ugly feeling and one that proves difficult to describe to anyone who doesn't have them. Friends I know who've been through it have said you don't know whether you are Arthur or Martha and that sometimes you're freezing and then moments later you're hot, hot, hot and wanting to strip bare.

My version of what happens during a hot flush is that the body produces estrogen and when a blocker, tamoxifen, is put in place, the brain really wants that estrogen because it needs it to do 'jobs', so there's conflict. The hot flush is the core of the argument – the clash of the disagreement, the epicentre of the war – and things just get explosive, hence the hot flush! My hot flushes would start in my toes, slowly rise through every cell of my body, forcing me to turn beetroot red, make me shift in my seat, sweat out of nowhere, kick off my shoes, take off a few layers and offer apologies to the company I kept. I would also learn to permanently have a bottle of water in my handbag.

From the standpoint of a cancer-risk perspective, I'm glad I had a mastectomy, but as the late, great Frank Sinatra once sang, 'Regrets, I've had a few...' I could never have entertained the idea of not ever doing it, however, now that it was done, I wish the outcome had have been different.

WHAT TO PACK FOR A MASTECTOMY SURGERY
- Tummy towel for the ride home
- Comfortable loose clothing
- Open front shirt/P.J.s
- Long phone lead for charger
- Own pillow if necessary
- Lip balm
- Bed socks
- Playlist
- Easy slip-on slippers
- Hand sanitiser
- Hairbrush (if you have hair)
- A 'blanky' (your favourite blanket for comfort)
- Lanyard – for drains

TOP TIPS
- Start the journey emotionally ready.
- Ask a lot of questions – I accepted what the doctors said and jumped in with both feet and had it done.
- Exercise lots for at least six months before your procedure and strengthen your core.
- Get multiple massages.

- Stay propped up.
- Use pillows at your side for your arms.
- Have two pillows under your knees, always.
- Have a travel pillow if you develop a hematoma/seroma.
- One-litre drink bottle – this ensures that you are staying hydrated a.m. and p.m.
- Seatbelt sleeve for travelling in the car (I had two – one for my car and one for John's car).
- An eye mask to block out the world if you want a day nap!
- Hand sanitiser for you and your visitors to prevent bugs and infection and to keep you as healthy as possible.
- Moisturiser to aid that lymph fluid to flow evenly around your body.
- Bed socks just because!
- A 'blanky' to relive your youth.
- Manicure, pedicure (no polish) and a haircut (it may be a while before you get to do that kind of thing).
- Postpone any appointments that require leaning backwards (dentist).
- Front button-up pyjamas.
- Front closure bra for easy access (if you can wear one).

Palpable lumps (lumps that can be felt) are often ignored and put down to other things such as mastitis (inflammation of a mammary gland), a lipoma (benign fatty tissue) or a fibroadenoma (benign growth). I have met many, many women who say they had a lump and did the unthinkable – they ignore it. We all know about lumps, but there are SO MANY MORE things to be aware of as potentially worrying signs – sore backs, a persistent cough, itchy breasts, a burning sensation, breasts sore to the touch, weight loss, piercing pains, pain in the shoulder, underarm pain, or one breast drooping lower than the other.

The international breast awareness campaign, 'Know Your Lemons', has found success using common fruit to make a statement about some of the signs and symptoms of this horrible disease.

'Until we find a cure for breast cancer, the best chance we have of survival is to find it as early as possible. For this to happen, we must be able to recognise the symptoms.'
Corrine Ellsworth Beaumont

SIGNS AND SYMPTOMS OF BREAST CANCER
- Thick mass
- Skin erosions
- Red or hot
- New fluid
- Dimpling
- Bump
- Growing vein
- Sunken nipple/nipple crusting
- New shape/size
- Orange peel skin
- Hard invisible lump

Visit www.*knowyourlemons.com* for further information. You could be delaying a diagnosis!

Humour and finding silver linings kept me going. I tapped into my DIEP social media group and there were nicknames for my newly-found status that were just hilarious. I couldn't believe how many there were:

Fatoobs (fat boobs), toobs (tummy boobs), stoobs (stomach boobs) floobs (flap boobs), reboobs (recycled boobs) and goobs (gut boobs).

In hindsight, I wish I would've been more proactive in preparation for such a big surgery. If I had my time again, I would've strengthened my core, stretched more using yin yoga and got myself as strong as I could. I wish I would've been more athletic. I wish I would've taken more time to decide to have DIEP – it was a rather quick decision and once I was committed, I didn't look back. I wish I would've had a little more clarity back then, but I was just so afraid. I thought by removing my breast tissue, skin and nipples, I would somehow feel and look abnormal.

Eleven

A bug's life

'It's okay to cry when there's too much on your mind
– the clouds rain too when things get heavy.'
Amina Mehmood

Hope had to be stronger than my fear.

I heard it before I saw it, like someone turning on a tap – not quite a flow, but not a drip either. On the floor were large droplets of fluid – not blood, but not clear. I couldn't work it out, but I knew it was mine. I stiffened, delicately lifting my gown where I could see fluid leaking from my left breast. It had soaked through my breast dressing and was unapologetically rolling down the arc of my breast and down my stomach.

I went through eight gowns over the next few hours. Each time I rose to move, it would ooze. It was sickening. A hematoma had burst inside my chest. For the next few weeks, I'd become very used to the same four hospital walls. The surgeries, chemotherapy and radiation had interrupted my life and my sleep, but what was to come would interrupt my physical being and try to bring me to my knees.

Wanting life to go to plan is all that anyone wants and it was definitely what I needed, but that simply wasn't meant to be. My utopian plan was to have a double mastectomy, recover, slowly gain my original strength and move on with my life.

My chest had not felt right after the DIEP procedure and the way it was looking was beginning to be confronting and scary. I began to notice that, instead of healing, the skin on my breasts and torso continued to feel extremely delicate and thin in places.

One month post-op, I began experiencing wounds (eruptions). There was a process. First, the dreaded pea-sized mark would appear on my breast, then I would watch this mark change in colour, but not in size, over about eight days. Like before, it would be followed by the slight peeling of the skin covering the wound, but revealing obvious fluid beneath. Seeing these 'holes' made me imagine an ant colony-style set-up inside my chest and I would experience a wave of nausea. My HITH (Hospital in the Home) nurse passively informed me that, 'These things track', as she placed the jumbo swab stick inside my chest to measure the depth of the eruption. This freaked me out and was never something that got easier. Once the wound was measured, it had to be 'packed'. It was a good job I wasn't squeamish because to some, this would be too much to bear! I could handle it. All those years of *Grey's Anatomy* had served me well!

Hanging on to my Civil Celebrancy course by a thread, I had spent hours making sure my latest wedding script was perfect and I was good to go. On the Saturday morning that I was due to present to my peers in class, I awoke to a damp feeling on my left side. Then I saw it. Immediately I knew that this definitely signalled the end of my course. I knew it was bad! I was on the hospital highway again, but this time, there was a bit more urgency behind it. (The six-month course eventually took me fifteen months, but I got there. Slow and steady, right?)

Concerned, HITH requested I be admitted to the hospital early December. I was told I would need a debridement surgery, as the sutures on my left breast had begun to show signs of opening. Debridement surgery is basically a good old cleanout. I was feeling really ill at this point. Mum and Dad, as usual, when they weren't managing our children, were beside me every moment of every day. Dad would bring me delicious salads to maintain my protein and promote healing, and Mum would keep my spirits up with her vivacious personality.

Kindness and thoughtfulness make a real difference when you are ill. This lifted my spirits and made me feel very loved. John had to explain to my family that I had to stay in the hospital for a little while longer and it was around this time that Layla and Lennox became a bit overwhelmed with all that was going on. I guess you could say they were just over it. Their school remained amazing and they set up an onsite counsellor who sent me pictures of activities they got up to at school, which was simply 'above and beyond.'

Debridement surgery number two was scheduled a few days after the initial one, as a yellow oily substance was oozing from my breast at this point. No prizes for guessing what that was. The doctors first thought was I was allergic to the anchor staples inside my chest post-op, but needed to 'go in' to fully investigate. Pathology was carried out during each operation, and it was strange to think that they were putting small parts of my body on petri dishes in multiple hospital laboratories in a city that I loved.

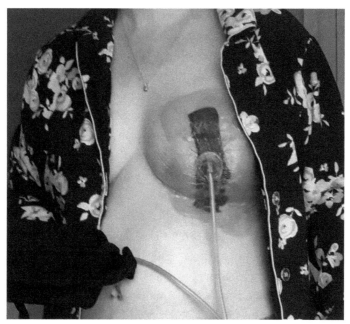

Me wearing one of two wound vacs.
It promotes quicker healing and drains at the same time.

I awoke with a wound vac attached to my breast. A wound vac is a bulky device that decreases air pressure on the wound, helping it to heal quicker from the inside out. A black sponge is placed with accuracy over the wound and a tube is attached to that and connected to the machine to create suction. It reminded me of when meat is vacuum-packed, but this time, it was happening on my chest. It wasn't a pain-free experience. The wound vac was to remain on for months and had to be changed regularly. During dressing changes (black sponge part), there were many apologies and, while the nurses told me to swear and let it all out, I didn't. Instead, I bit down on my gown and attempted to find my happy place which, at that point, was a swimming pool full of painkillers!

The next twelve months was all about interruption and eruptions. My stomach was beginning to show very ugly signs of breaking down before my eyes and everyone involved was fairly worried. Running parallel to this, I was managing the 'pimple' which was worsening at the back of my head by the day. It became very oozy and, as horrible as this may sound, when I would pull at it, gatherings of hair would come out with small chunks of flesh attached, making me realise that parts of my scalp were coming off! It did leave a small crater at the back of my head and took nearly a year to heal. I now have a small bald patch that is easily covered by my curls, which is great.

Watching my breast wound open minute by minute is the strangest thing and it nearly pushed me over the edge. A young surgeon who knew about my situation, stopped, pulled up a chair and chatted to me for a while. She was awesome and told me to write the day off as a bad health day. I immediately felt better. I will never forget that young surgeon with her tender bedside manner. At this stage, the doctors deemed it strange for the eruptions to transfer from one breast to the other and even stranger when it transferred to my stomach. No amount of sleep could have prepared me for what happened next.

I was moments away from the porter arriving for debridement surgery number three when in walked my team of surgeons, flanked with students. They had a spring in their step and smiles on their faces. 'We've found out what's wrong with you. We worked it out', they were exclaiming. Wait, what? There's something wrong with me? Wrong. That word bounced around my head in slow motion. Something else? There has *been* something wrong with me already and I had that removed in February! It's supposed to be over. I'm scrambling to get my life back here!

Mum and Dad edged forward on their seats. The specialists went on to reveal that I had a rather nasty bacteria inside my body. Its name was *mycobacterium fortuitum*. This is a bacteria known to cause infections in many areas of the body, including the skin. It can be found in water, sewage, dirt and surgical equipment. Normally, healthy people don't get this type of infection. However, due to my immune system being impaired, I was left open to infection and had been for a while.

The anchor staple allergy theory was put to bed and a plan had to be quickly made. They needed to get me on some serious, heavy-duty medication and fast. Having my mum with me, especially when a specialist came to visit, was invaluable. She absorbed every spoken word, not missing a thing. She behaved like a human dictaphone and became expert at replaying relevant conversations as we tried to unravel what all this meant for me, the future and my family's future! 'It's a skill,' she told me – a skill that currently I was unable to tap into, damn chemo fog!

Oh my. A bacteria had grown inside me! My stomach dropped when I heard that news. What the actual hell????? There was something in my body that was very complicated and complex, but there was no way I was going to take this lying down. In saying that, my worries magnified when I was told that this bacteria was so rare, it was maybe only seen once a year in Australia. Hello, I was their 2018 model! Questions whizzed through my mind and Mum and Dad were left speechless.

I was whisked away by a porter and found myself calling over my shoulder, 'Google it, mum, Google what the hell it is.' There was simply no time to ask any questions. It was bad timing and I was left to process this latest disaster on the operating table! Hoping my inner strength would prevail, my mind worked hard to overcome the feeling of being overwhelmed. Realising I'd forgotten to ask if what I had was dangerous, deadly even, left me feeling worried. Things had just gone in a very different direction. I was stressed out and could feel my sunflower petals falling off. Being thrown into a world that I knew nothing about was not on my agenda.

It was December 3rd, 2018. This was the time when I started to think I definitely had a story to tell, something to pen. I was being tested by life now and it was truly daunting. Previously, I had been able to see cancer on an ultrasound and trace my finger over my stomach and breast scars, but *mycobacterium fortuitum* remained elusive and sneaky and, frankly, hard to kill. The bacteria turned out to be relentless. It was a rotten, stinking setback and I was left disappointed by life once again.

Clinical walls became home, complete with the constant flow of pills in cups. I craved John's company, but had to settle with infrequent bed dates. John would send me messages with pictures of himself and our children doing various activities, and while the sentiment was appreciated and I wouldn't have had it any other way, once in a while it would make me feel down because I missed them so deeply.

In the hospital, I felt absent from my own life. This was a stark contrast to the life I was used to and sometimes I felt as if I was going insane from boredom. I had to cheer up. I began relaxing to the sweet sounds of different musical artists from my day. Replaying these songs helped me realise what a fantastic life I had been blessed with as each familiar track formed a lovely memory. The next day, Layla called me with great news. She had been awarded the role of school captain. My tears were a blend of joy with a sprinkle of sadness because I could not cuddle her, swing her around, tickle her and unleash an embarrassing amount of kisses upon her. I was so proud and it helped me turn a corner that day.

A further debridement and washout were required to get rid of all the necrosis (the death of cells and tissue) happening inside the left breast. Necrosis happened to me because many of the cells in the transplanted tissue died because of the bacteria feasting on it. It makes me queasy to think about it like that.

During that operation, it was decided that I would have some stitches to fix up my stomach and another fairly decent-sized hole above the nipple on my left breast too. Layla and Lennox were desperate to see me, but we didn't want to stress them out or cause any unnecessary worry. I was fitted with a second wound vac because of my stomach wound. I wasn't in a good way and John and I didn't want our children to see me in such a vulnerable state. When they did visit, hopping into bed with me was something that we all enjoyed. Layla snuggled in close and was a bit heartbroken while I could hear Lennox doing loud, exaggerated martial arts moves in the corridor. Such chalk and cheese!

As if receiving news that I had a strain of the flesh-eating bacteria wasn't shocking enough, I was about to be emotionally tested. My parents made their usual trip down the hospital highway, but arrived looking forlorn. Something was wrong. My cousin, Clare, who lives in Belfast, Northern Ireland, had lost her seventeen year-old son, Seamus, the night before. He was her second son, one of five boys, and this desperate upset was to ricochet through our family for a long time. The news was trying to threaten my rock-solid attitude and crying myself to sleep that night made me think how cruel life was that we couldn't make it to his funeral. I also felt guilty that my poor parents could not be there because they were too busy tied up with me!

The morning saw no less heartbreak. I woke with tears in my eyes. I spent the day sobbing on and off to the point where the nursing staff sent me a hospital counsellor as they knew some of my tears were about Seamus, but there were probably some underlying issues too. The impact of treatment on my capacity to work, perform activities and drive were heightened. It felt good to openly cry. I felt entitled to. My life had been totally disrupted and I was walking down roads I didn't want to. I let it all out that day and my heart was broken for Clare and my extended family members.

Mum and Dad relayed the sad news to John and the children once they were home. Later that evening, I received a picture message. Lennox had written, '*My heart beats for you*' on a post-it note. I was just thrilled and felt proud that we were in tune with each other. He knows that I'm a softy and that the news of Seamus would've caused me heartache and pain. What he also knew in his nine-year-old beating heart is that Mummy would really have needed that post-it note. Not long after, Layla wrote me a message on a love heart note which read, '*Keep fighting*'. Such notes had impact and I loved the feeling of that organic support.

Post-chemotherapy, my internal microbiome (something in the gut that protects us against germs) was about to be subjected to total deforestation. My gut flora had already been through the wringer and now I needed to take medication as *Mycobacterium fortuitum* can cause infections in the skin, lymph nodes and joints.

My medical status at the time meant that I was under the oncology plastics department of the hospital. To add to that, I was now referred to the Infectious Disease Department. Two departments! I was supposed to be taking baby steps forward, not giant leaps backwards. Two very pleasant infectious disease doctors arrived and prescribed an avalanche of antibiotics. Over the next gruelling eight-and-a-half months, I was to swallow multiple pills in a bid to prevent my chest from being eaten alive.

Due to my new situation, and after some serious consideration, we decided to forfeit a rural holiday we had booked to Cohuna, Victoria. It wasn't going to work as I was simply not well enough. It was only day five of these strong tablets and I was not feeling great. We decided that we would book a fabulous family holiday, just the four of us, when this nightmare was all over. It was upsetting to have to cancel yet another break due to my ill health and I felt angry and disappointed. It was to take a further eleven months before we were to travel to the Cook Islands and have a week of pure bliss, time to connect, and a whole lot of fun.

After this discharge from the hospital, I stopped off to pick up a Sunday-to-Monday pillbox which left me feeling rather like a nanna, but after only a week of pill popping, I was re-admitted to the hospital. Once again, I was taken into theatre for another debridement and washout. By this point, the suture line running from the bottom of my left nipple to under the breast was completely open, revealing the transplanted tissue underneath. It was watermelon red and looked angry and bumpy. The surgeons kept reassuring me they were extremely happy with what they saw and explained that, even though I could see a huge area of the inside of my breast from the outside, they knew it was red, healthy and clean. There was no need for alarm, but it would prove impossible to be 'pulled' back together.

– WARNING GRAPHIC CONTENT NEXT PAGE –

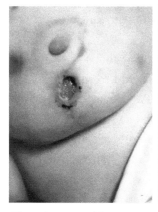 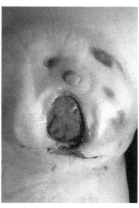

Eruptions would appear every third day.   *Early stages of damage.*

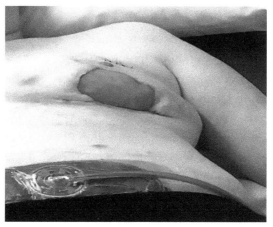

Picture taken during a dressing change of the wound vac.
Note the stomach wound vac…… double trouble!

A further debridement and washout showed some progressive healing and there was talk of a skin graft operation in the New Year. This was positive news. The wound vac was working and I was hoping to get home for Christmas. A dent in my armour saw me wake from my last debridement surgery with not one, but two wound vacs – one on my breast and the other on my stomach! Merry bloody Christmas!

I surprised Layla and Lennox by returning home six days before Santa was due, and things were going great. Channel 7 had been in touch again, asking to do a follow-up on my health. I thought it strange as things were fairly quiet with me. Then, a deliriously magical thing happened.

ROISIN:

'After a year of my sister and I being battered from chemotherapy and having multiple surgeries, Michael, Ivy and I surprised her by making the long journey to Australia for that hug we have both been so desperate for. It was the best feeling on earth.'

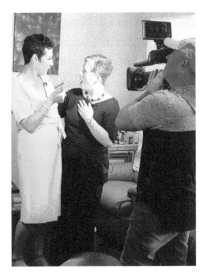 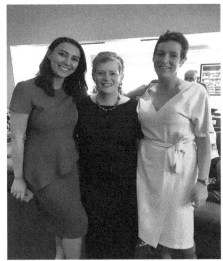

Roisin surprises me by flying over from England with her family (left). Estelle Griepink, journalist from Channel 7 with myself (middle) and Roisin. December 2019.

I was in shock! Believing that Channel 7 were in my home that afternoon simply to do a follow-up was completely feasible to me but, really, they were all in on the reunion too. I was elated and knew it was going to be a great Christmas. Once again we made the news both here in Australia and over in the U.K., and even gave the Queen's speech a run for her money with all the 'hits' we got on the internet!

My elation, while sweet, didn't last. I had a serious bleed again and HITH assessed me and deemed me too sick to be at home. So, on Christmas Eve they placed me in the Emergency Department once again. The nurses looking after me were amazing, but my body just wasn't playing the game.

Being in hospital for Christmas did not feel right at all. Having the ultimate party for one was not what I had planned. I had to 'prison break'. I was nicknamed 'the energiser bunny' as I usually run rings around my peers when it comes to daily duties, but my stamina had abandoned me. I'd hit a brick wall. I was experiencing exhaustion and my body was limp.

As the days rolled into each other I learned what my capabilities were, and the list wasn't that long. I have never been a lazy person so the forced rest and recuperation, especially at Christmas, was pretty tough mentally. I had to accept that my body was trying to reboot itself and that when I was resting, I wasn't wasting time: I was recovering. I was told off ALL the time by many for saying sentences prefaced with, 'Sorry'. Sorry, I can't help. Sorry I can't drive the children to school. Sorry I can't stay awake for that family movie. Sorry I can't wash my hair. Sorry, sorry, sorry. Sigh! It felt foreign, but I knew it was necessary. Eventually, I embraced the rest and recovery. What I didn't realise was how long this recovery was going to be.

After hefty persuasion on my part, I managed to be discharged the night of Christmas Eve around eight o'clock with a promise of return three days later. All was good with the world. I had a wonderful Christmas Day because it was filled with family, food and fun. The best part was I didn't, for the first time in a long time, have to do anything at all. My little elves were Christmas experts.

At bedtime, Lennox entered our bedroom just as I was getting into my pyjamas. He remarked that my fifty-two-centimetre abdominal scar looked like I had been sawn in half as magicians did on television. Amused, I decided that was going to be my story if anyone ever asked me about how I came to have the scar on my stomach. At that moment, I loved that we could laugh about something so horrible. As he left the room, I started thinking about Lennox and Layla and what they might look like on their wedding days. I immediately burst into tears and found myself hoping I'd be alive for them. That bloody pendulum, always swinging at random times.

As promised, I was back in the hospital and Bed 12 had become my safe place. The staff kept giving me the same room and nicknamed me 'The Frequent Flyer.' Here I had no responsibilities other than to myself. I became frustrated that my sister and her family had come over to see me and I had hardly been home. I was finally discharged, this time on New Year's Eve, which was great. As a family, we all sat around on the decking, me with my water, pills and wound vacs, and the rest of my family drinking wine. I couldn't bring myself to sulk; I was just grateful to be alive, to be home and to be sitting with my people.

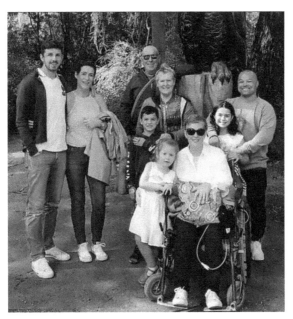

My home office photo. All of us visiting Healesville
Sanctuary, Melbourne in 2019.

Spending so much time in hospital while my U.K. family were in Australia made me crave a family day out. Roisin going home was creeping up fast. We settled on Healesville Sanctuary, a zoo specialising in native Australian animals. It was perfect for all my visitors. A photograph was captured that day that I now have in my office and I look at most days. Replaying the laughs and shenanigans of the day brings me such warmth.

The time had come for Roisin, her husband Michael Brown, and Ivy to leave Melbourne and make the long-haul flight back to England. It was just awful. There were many tears and lots of hugs, but our worlds were forever improved because of their visit. My parents were with us for five more precious days.

Once I was allowed to shower again, it became exhausting both physically and mentally, as it became the crying chamber again when things just got a little too much. Once again to appease the children, I pretended to get shampoo in my eyes. I felt terrible that my sister was going home to lifelong chemotherapy while I was dealing with this crap at the same time. The awful bacteria episode had, once again, left me feeling betrayed by my own body.

The Infectious Disease Department changed tactic and brought out the pharmaceutical big guns. I was placed on a strong antibiotic that needed to be administered 24/7 via a PICC line. Similar to a catheter, it would be put in on the inside of my left arm and dropped into my heart.

This new medication was attached to a container called a 'Baxter' that looked like a baby's bottle and rested in a very undesirable bum bag that followed me everywhere! That thing was annoying and I had to be on high alert because I did get Baxter caught on several door handles during our time together. The idea of it ripping out of my heart was just too much to bear. I became vigilant with it but it was definitely a bad fashion statement. Another medication, Amikacin, was provided through a drip and brought with it fatigue and accumulative vertigo. That was it. After ten days, I was taken off it. Vertigo is awful and the doctors had to go to Plan B, which was pills, pills and more pills!

I was eventually told that I could cease medications to treat the bacteria. It had been months and months of internal hell and I squealed and hugged my doctor at the good news. He was all smiles and I couldn't wait to put this nightmare behind me and move forward. Hoping that one day I could have corrective surgery made me upbeat and I couldn't wait to go home and tell my family. I remained hopeful about re-reconstruction in my future and this made me walk that bit taller.

Twelve

Correction

*'It's like a never-ending story. If you are not preparing for
upcoming tests, you are always talking about your cancer to
people. When you are not talking about it, you're thinking
about it and when you're not trying to think about it, you feel a
pain, get a scare and find yourself thinking about it again!'*
B.J. – cancer survivor

When I think of my body, sometimes sadness still grips me.
It wraps its arms around me and squeezes.

Discretion had abandoned ship with any medical professionals at this
point. I had become a total over-sharer, offering anyone who would look
a glance at my chest. I continue to remain 'on guard' when it comes to not
ignoring niggles or twinges, no matter how small. I often find myself staring
into my full-length mirror surveying the damage. Touching my breasts took
me an eternity. They did, and still do, feel broken and foreign to me. I walk
the earth, knowing the horror under my shirt.

I had wound dressings on my chest for 332 days in total. That's nearly a
year of worrying whether it had soaked through my outfit and wondering
how long this eruption would take to close… wondering if I would ever
wear a nice bra again or be well enough to work. While examining myself,
I was very aware of the numbness. This was to be expected from the type of
surgery undertaken. John very cheekily asked if I'd like some help checking
for numb areas. I had to warn him that it would be pointless and that I
probably wouldn't feel a thing. He convinced himself in that moment that

he had 'magic hands' and he bet me fifty dollars that he could make me feel his touch. He lost. It was total bullshit. I silently screamed at the universe to stop holding me back.

It was time for another difficult goodbye. My parents had to jetset back home to continue to support Roisin with her ongoing cancer-kicking battle. As Dad and I embraced, the world slowed down momentarily and he whispered, 'Every room is brighter because you are in it.' It broke my heart because I wanted to be in every room with him and Mum for so much longer. I took to wearing my dad's 'aftershave-coated' hoodie that he had left in my car and, like a baby's blanky, it brought me endless comfort.

MUM:

'Leaving to return to the U.K. was one of the hardest things we have ever had to do as parents and our tears flowed all the way back to England.'

My mother-in-law, also from the U.K., arrived twenty-four hours after my parents left. She, too, blessed us with a helping hand and it made this phase of my recovery very easy.

January 2019 saw my year start with a skin graft from my left leg to finally close the hole in my breast, which, by this point, was pushing ten centimetres. It all went without a hitch, leaving us all relieved. Previously, my world had shrunk when I was confined to the chemo chair. I became Jeff Jefferies in the Alfred Hitchcock movie, *Rear Window*, so now that I was 'making lemonade', I decided to get out and about a bit more.

Thoughts of bra shopping were reeling me in. People who have my kind of surgery are encouraged to wear bras with no underwire. The reasoning is quite hideous! If the underwire came loose and poked me, there's a chance I wouldn't be able to feel it due to reduced sensitivity. There were horror stories of women being impaled in the breast with underwire and I found it just so weird! Ultimately, what seemed like a good idea soon turned into a BAD idea. When shopping, nothing seemed to fit, look right or feel right. Even shopping for tops and dresses had become difficult and, with not having to worry about the bust size now, things just sat wrong. Stressed, I left empty-handed. I had to work hard to remind myself that I preferred this banged-up body over the alternative. I was with Mandy and she suggested a glass of bubbles. That made the pity party I was having come to a screeching halt. Things could be so much worse and I just needed to get on because I was a beautiful survivor!

Appointments every forty-eight hours with my G.P. and the nurses for my wound care became ongoing. It was like *Groundhog Day*. On day one of wound care at the G.P.'s clinic, one of the secretaries who knew me well, saw me and, with a shocked look, enquired if I was okay. She replied by telling me that she wondered where I had been. 'One minute you are here and next you fell off our radar'. I asked, 'Did you think I was dead?' She laughed hysterically and I knew that she had been thinking that. I assured her I was going nowhere.

Of course, there were times where I would cry and be sad, but relying on my inner strength to prevail was the only way. When I did have a 'moment', I chose to acknowledge it and then try to understand it. Why was I feeling this? The answer is always the same: it is chaos and fear. Nearly all of the time, it's because of something connected to Layla and Lennox. Like the time when I walked to the mailbox from my front door and inside was a parcel. I knew what it was – a birthday book for my son from his Grandma. As I touched it, sinister thoughts of not being around for future birthdays went through me like an electric shock. I hated the fact that I mightn't know what our children would look like when they're older. Bad thoughts flooded me and, before I knew it, I was inside the house quietly sobbing with my hand covering my mouth. The mirror in the lounge room caught my reflection and I stopped myself. My pain did not last as long, because I was able to acknowledge that I was scared. I was scared, and that was okay because cancer is scary. These events often caught me off guard and they were not pleasant but I knew how to push back and beat the tears.

Then… Dear Lindsey, I have another gift for you from cancer.

My breast surgeon was concerned I had developed cording, and referred me to a local specialist named Jenny for advice and treatment. Cording is like having a rope-like structure pulled taut underneath your flesh that starts mainly in the armpit, then embeds itself in the breast and travels down the arm, preventing it from being fully straightened. Luckily, I only dealt with cording for a short time and saw it mainly as an inconvenience, but I could physically see the raised cord in my arm and it was unsettling. I was advised that popping the cording through self-massage would offer instant relief and I was up for it. I knew it would take a while, but, with patience, I was hoping for it to organically resolve itself. Sure enough, after persistent manipulation by yours truly, the cording popped painlessly and I was all fixed.

During my first appointment, Jenny asked to inspect my torso. She witnessed the unsavoury secrets underneath my clothes, but it was business as usual and I was getting out my boobs to a specialist once again. She held a strong but empathetic gaze as she enquired about what had been going on for me to have ended up looking like I did. Not only were my breasts looking damaged, but my stomach also looked like I had swallowed a basketball, something that had started since the day I woke up from my DIEP procedure. I told her that some specialists had said, reassuringly, that because I contracted the bacteria, my body had prioritised which problem to solve first and it had chosen the bacteria.

Shortly after, Jenny informed me that she strongly believed I had truncal lymphoedema or 'swelly belly' as it is nicknamed. Fabulous! Who knew there could be so many gifts? Was there a Guinness world record for someone who could have so many things go wrong when they are diagnosed with breast cancer? If so, I was a strong contender for the main prize.

Lymphoedema is a side effect of my cancer treatment and very annoying to be honest. Peering down at my rather portly distended 'swelly belly' is a daily reminder of what has happened to me. The sensation of numbness is something I'm still not used to and the worst part is that I can never tell if my pants are falling down because I can't feel it! John lovingly joked that I was Budda minus the wisdom. I wonder if I rub it enough, will it bring me good luck?

Truncal lymphedema across the waistline is directly linked to stomach trauma. I had to wear a binder that was hot and hard. It pulled my stomach in, but it also cut in at the waist, gave me very unattractive back fat and was stiff, oh so stiff. A small, peach sponge pad with bobbles on it was placed in my underwear at the front just to add to the attraction, deterring the pooling effect of the lymphatic fluid. It left a mark on my lower stomach in the groin area and Lennox and Layla thought this to be rather hilarious. Lennox dropped to his knees and pretended to type on the 'keyboard' and Layla acted out a game of Connect 4 as the impressions of the bobbles became entertainment for them. I had a newfound respect for the corset-wearing Victorians! Previously my old stomach had been malleable and warm, similar to Play-Doh and now it was swollen, hard, numb and tight! I wondered how long it would take to feel normal.

Around eighteen months post-DIEP, I began to experience a feeling of painless, but strikingly obvious movement across the inside my abdomen – a definite rolling and pulling sensation. It resembled the feeling of being six to eight months pregnant. It was very strange and felt as if there was a baby in there moving from side to side. It reminded me of the movie, *Alien,* because I was CERTAIN I was not expecting. I couldn't be pregnant – we had managed that situation by vasectomy in 2010! As quickly as it arrived, it left, and that is just about the weirdest thing that happened to me during my whole cancer experience.

It was early August 2019 when I heard that my plastic surgeon was changing hospitals. The transient state of the medical world meant that I'd be assigned a new plastic surgeon. This was unnerving, but a fresh set of eyes was maybe what I needed. I prayed that the new guy was just as much as a perfectionist as my previous one. With new surgeons come new ideas, new strategies, new approaches and, most importantly, new conversation.

At the end of that month, I made a decision. If I wanted to maximise life's full potential, I knew I had to move more, so with Martine's persistent encouragement, I joined a gym. I didn't fight for my life just to stop living. I needed – not wanted, *needed* – to exercise the past away… to reshape my mind, body and soul. At first, I was averse to it. Breathing other people's sweat in a room was not my idea of health, but it has turned out to be the best thing I could've done. Firstly, it gave me endorphins, then, by attending yoga classes, I began to break down some physical stiffness. Going to the gym allowed me to regain a sense of new normality and I saw it as being kind to myself.

The Little Things

One morning I was busy annihilating fat cells on the torturous but strangely satisfying StairMaster when out of the corner of my eye I saw an abandoned 'Genesis Care' drink bottle. Whilst I had been blessed with a good experience with Genesis care as you have read, I was not about to let it invade my personal space when I am trying damn hard to move on. I started irrationally and silently arguing with the bottle in my head. What are you doing here? What the hell? Go away, you are not allowed to be here. I'm done with you. Stop hindering my recovery. Bugger off. I caught myself looking at it with total disapproval, followed by forcing myself to stop mentally telling off a bit of plastic on top of the gym drink tower.

I remained hopeful for a scan and for someone to say, 'Lindsey, there is no evidence of disease (NED).' During my appointments, my breast surgeon always seemed so stoic and professional. One day I ran my eyes over her side profile as she typed, and pondered over how many hours she had spent doing surgeries over the last week, how many hours she'd been in the car driving between multiple hospitals, how many meetings she'd attended or whether there had been any emergencies. She knew all my struggles about all the intimate parts of my body, yet I knew nothing of her. Isn't it funny what you think about during appointments?

(These days, I'm still being monitored by the specialist every six months, with intense breast checks.)

Now, hadn't cancer taken enough? Here I sat with no sexual feelings or urges (thanks, tamoxifen) and a downstairs love area that felt like the Kalahari Desert. There was only one cream I knew of that was supposed to help with my lady bits and I was allergic to it… of course I was! However, dig a bit deeper and I found a tip that promotes using coconut oil formed with a melon baller and then put in the freezer to alleviate discomfort. Really? I didn't know whether to laugh or cry. Have I tried it yet? No. Will I? No.

Would we ever get those glory years back in the bedroom? It's a secret! Realistically, I knew that one day it would be back. I was too young for this and no matter how long it took, John always reassured me that it was all going to be okay. We shared evolving vocabulary about what mattered. Over the last two years, physical changes were obvious, mental challenges were real and we both, at times, moved between feeling on top of things (pun intended) and thinking, *What the hell is happening to us?*

Losing weight had begun, and I was also seeing a naturopath to rebuild my gut health and was getting stronger every day. By the end of 2019, I was beginning to feel proud of my body, how it was beginning to look and how it had coped. Feeling physically stronger meant that bonding with John was seriously worth waiting for (*wink, wink*). When we were young, I used to get butterflies knowing that I would see him soon and before we knew it, 'life' happened: mortgages, children, careers… and things slowed down. Now it is a beautiful relationship and I can honestly say I love him more each day. Even the butterflies have a flutter now and again. I don't doubt in my mind that we will always walk together and be stronger for it. Whether what has happened to us is a curse or a gift, who knows. I just know I'm damn lucky to have him by my side.

When sharing my sister's story about her first diagnosis – the one where she's pregnant – I used to refer to her as a 'breast cancer survivor'. In my head, I thought this was simply that she had breast cancer and now she doesn't. Now, after walking the same path, the word 'survivor' is not strong enough. The mental torture that you go through at times can be overwhelming. We both agree it's unhealthy to look backwards and think, *If only,* or *What if I just went flat,* or the *Should've done this* approach, but often these thoughts just take over and that fierce, strong mindset that we have inside us pushes through and calms the storm.

January 2020 saw my non-cancerous left breast begin the long journey of being rebuilt for the second time. I had a LICAP (lateral intercostal artery perforator) flap reconstruction procedure, which would see redundant fatty tissue being used to replace missing breast tissue and, as much as possible, restore it to its normal size and shape. It would take approximately three surgeries, the first being the flap transplant, the others fat grafting. This would give me shape and contour. It was my tenth operation, which, unfortunately, clashed with our sixteenth wedding anniversary. The surgery went without a hitch and I was discharged two days later on my forty-sixth birthday.

Healing was slow, but I was driving after five days and out and about after ten. Lennox took to measuring my scars – it was his inner Jack Sparrow! He let us all know it was a 'whopping twenty-six centimetres' (his words). It was exactly half the size of the one on my stomach. My scars represented cancer's curse and hardship and were an outward representation of the inward battle I faced. However, this did not make looking at them any easier.

Thirteen

Bits of me in the bin

'I will always appreciate the small things: I will kick up my heels, I will have my cake and eat it, I will make a difference in someone's day, I will find my mantra, I will act like a kid occasionally, I will be empathetic, I will enjoy a belly laugh or two, I will celebrate life, I will keep learning, I will take the time to reflect, I will tackle life head-on, I will explore more, I will smile more.'
Wallpaper quotes – anonymous

I was scheduled to have a partial hysterectomy, which had been recommended by my oncologist. The removal of my ovaries and fallopian tubes had been part of my cancer plan right from the start, when my cancer was found to be ER+ (estrogen receptor-positive, meaning the estrogen had been feeding my original tumour). It had just taken a while to get there because of all the medical complications. It seemed silly, but I was excited about this. Previously, I would never have been excited about surgery but for me, this was another step towards hopefully never getting cancer again.

Removing both ovaries was two-fold: it could help prevent ovarian cancer in the future, and stop the major source of estrogen production in my body. Tamoxifen would also be stopped and I would be placed on another aromatase inhibitor – a type of hormone therapy for postmenopausal women. I turned into a giggly teenager on a first date at the mere idea of giving up tamoxifen.

I met with my oncologist who referred me to a gynaecologist who would whip part of my baby-making equipment out. Breast procedures had been my reality for quite some time and the fact that another part of my woman-hood was about to be tossed out hit home. I was excited, but sad at the same time.

The gynaecologist I saw was brilliant. She thought fast, talked fast and put a plan together fast, all while making me feel totally at ease and able to ask any questions. My wait for a surgery date wasn't too long. It was scheduled for the day after the first anniversary of my double mastectomy, a slap-in-the-face reminder of just how long I'd been dealing with this cancer crap!

My surgery had the funniest name. It was called a laparoscopic bilateral salpingo-oophorectomy.

> **Laparoscopic:** *minimally invasive*
> **Bilateral:** *both sides*
> **Salpingo:** *fallopian tube removal*
> **Oophorectomy** *(pronounced oof-er-ec-tomy): ovary removal*

To me, it sounded like the name of a Mexican block of flats and made me amused whenever I heard it.

Layla had been at school camp and was due back late afternoon on the day of my surgery. She had expressed a bit of concern that she wasn't going to see me the morning of my procedure to wish me good luck. Knowing that John and I were raising such an empathetic young woman was a great feeling.

John and Lennox drove me to the hospital. After the all-too-familiar check-in, I met with the nurse to go over my health history and we both agreed it was fairly extensive. Next, it was time to dress for surgery. The dressing gown, white gown, hair net and the booties were all given to me like an inmate receiving their uniform. John had to assist putting the compression socks on as I still found it awkward to engage my core and fully fold in half post-DIEP. We sat quietly watching old re-runs of shows from the nineties that were doing their job of removing us from reality.

I sent John home because the sound of his stomach rumbling was making me hungry. Being wheeled into the operating room, the distinctive coldness of the room hit me. I began to get creative – this time, when the piranha effect was happening, I imagined I was a fashion model in Milan getting 'spruced'. It was show time. I was hooked up, wired up and ready for sleep. I knew this surgery was not to be underestimated. I was going to be classed as 'in menopause' in the next two hours and that, to me, was a big deal. The sleepy face mask was placed over my face and I began my long, slow, deep breaths. It was lights out fairly quickly. I was under for less than two hours.

My excitement to stop tamoxifen was short-lived. After only a one-night stay, the discharging nurses informed me that I had to keep taking it until I had seen my oncologist, which was scheduled for twelve days later. Like a naughty child, I tutted under my breath and I was mentally on countdown. I left praying for a favourable pathology result.

At home, I knew to expect less energy than usual and a bit of pain. I was only taking over-the-counter painkillers and was comfortable with that. In previous surgeries, I would often feel guilty and try to at least get out of bed and help around the house, but John had time off and this allowed me to surrender to the effects of the operation. Once again, I operated in nanna mode with slippers and energy levels to match, but good sleep and rest were essential to my recovery. I already missed the gym and found myself thinking about what kind of modified program they would put me on upon my return. Friends dropped in and, once again, the love around me ramped up, making me nothing but happy.

May I once again be allowed to talk all things bowels for a moment? This is one area during treatment that has the potential to send me crazy. I had never suffered constipation throughout my whole life even during chemotherapy – never, never, ever until this point. Goodness gracious me. Both Sean and Roisin had struggled and had told me that constipation was one of the worst parts of a diagnosis. For me, holding a 'seated toilet position' for forty-five minutes was a challenge. I had given myself a half-time break at one point to go and get my phone. *What?* I was bored in there and needed the distraction. Having my handset in the bathroom was not common practice with me, but, desperate times called for desperate measures. After a while, I caved and sent Martine an S.O.S. call to please bring me liquorice.

A natural heat pack, pain medication, the chemo chair, water, snacks and Netflix eased any discomfort for me in those first few days and then, each day saw me get stronger and stronger. Day three saw me dress in very loose-fitting clothes and my family fuss over me whenever there was eye contact. Layla caught me popping something in the dishwasher and with a louder voice than normal exclaimed, 'Mum, stop bending down.' I told her I wanted to be a bit more active. She vehemently disagreed. 'Just because you look better, it does not mean that the inside of your tummy is better.' I satisfied her by returning to my chemo chair – pronto.

With my ovaries and fallopian tubes now in the bin, I knew I had to change medications. Starting any new drug is mostly a mental game. After a meeting with my oncologist, my new medication was called anastrozole. When thinking about anastrozole, the benefit for me had to outweigh the risk. I had no fear whatsoever of the side effects that might come with taking it. None, zilch, nada. I had to rely on its effectiveness in preventing a breast cancer recurrence and just swallow the damn thing. I needed to give my family their wife and mum back.

I remember talking to anastrozole. Before I swallowed the little white pill, I requested it to treat me well. In the early days and all for free, anastrozole came with the inability to do homework with our children (especially maths), a free tropical holiday on my face (the ever-so-unpredictable hot flush), and a temper that saw me growl like a bear. I also mimicked Dory from 'Finding Nemo' with my short-term memory loss and it was all very frustrating. I cursed that four-centimetre tumour most days and was generally an all-round cranky pants. I watched our children's faces change under my constant lectures. They looked at me in bewilderment. I could hear myself speaking out of character and wanted to stop but just couldn't. Behaving like this was not something I did. The number of iPad bans I was handing out was incredible. I knew something was wrong.

I checked in on myself during a meditation class at the gym and decided a change was due. I was angry on anastrozole and the bear had to go. Giving John the anastrozole side-effects sheet was a bid to work through this adjustment together. I had turned into a madwoman and didn't want to stress him out. I apologised to everyone and felt guilty and dramatic. I explained that it would seem I was in anastrozole's control… for now.

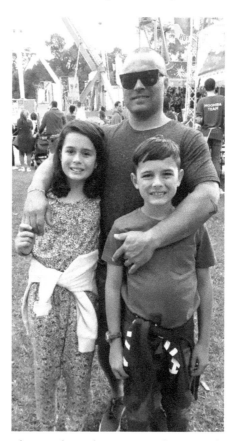

John, Layla and Lennox at the Moomba
Festival in Melbourne, Australia March 2019.

Things did get easier as the chemical found its place in its new habitat and the placebo effect delivered a sense of calm. My sleep drastically improved, but the health of my feet and ankles was somewhat compromised. As explained by the oncologist, achy feet and ankles are a textbook side effect of the drug. On the bad nights, I would stare at John as he slept, desperately wanting to shake him and say, 'Help me John, help me manage myself.' That's how fraught you can feel. Of course, I didn't. He was the only one earning any money in the house and I needed to respect that by letting him sleep.

I was left wondering if I'd become half-bloke now. After all, I had no ovaries, no fallopian tubes and no breasts! I felt assaulted by life and I could not wait to get back to the gym for my daily injections of endorphins. This was menopause, God-damned menopause. I had been here before. I had gone through chemical menopause with chemotherapy, then medical menopause with the tamoxifen, and now surgically-induced menopause. I thought about whether I would have natural menopause when I was off the anastrozole. That is a lot of menopauses for one little lady! Somebody pass me a cold compress and open a window!

Fourteen

Acts of kindness

'Try to be a rainbow in someone's cloud.'
Maya Angelou

'I just don't know how to help.' 'I don't know what to say.' It's been so long with an extensive list of treatments with many twists and turns, but my friends and family have never skipped a beat. The stream of support has been endless. I've been spoilt at many lunches, had pedicures, had meal plans put together in and around my surgeries, and they have babysat our children at a moment's notice. They have taken me to appointments and kept me laughing the whole way. Knowing the ripple effect that cancer can create, they've cared not only for me, but John and our children too. They have been there since day one, always ready to add another layer of fighting talk, and they've epitomised the spirit of love and kindness. Their positive words have made having cancer a lot easier than I thought it would be.

There have been so many lovely moments – too many to mention – but I would love to share some with you. You never know, this may help you get ideas for your future friends because unfortunately, statistically, the number of people diagnosed with cancer is rising – not falling – and having support is vital. It makes you feel as if you can conquer anything.

One of the best visits was from a lady I knew through work who turned up with twelve organic eggs, plain Greek yoghurt and a bag of fresh fruit. Brilliant! She said, 'I didn't know what to get and I knew you had to eat well, so I brought you food.' I loved it! I have also received the best practical gifts, such as fuzzy bed socks, relaxing colouring books, hand cream, aluminium-free deodorant, face masks (genius), blankets, art books, guardian angel pins, a comfortable robe, icy poles for when the metallic taste was there, and extra soft toothbrushes.

All this support meant that my family and friends created a warm environment which helped me manage the 'tumble dryer' effect I was experiencing. I promised I would always be open to conversation, honest about how I was feeling and would never fake-smile. If I was having a bad day, my 'village' would know about it. I aired all my laundry, scars and all.

Cancer truly has a ripple effect; I honestly believe that what happened to me, happened to us all. I was lucky enough to have a loving, committed group of people behind me who drove my positivity to its full potential. My positive attitude acted partly as my medicine, I suppose; it gave me strength. Mentally, this was scary stuff at times, but I knew where to go when I needed support. I had people posting things in the mail and online that offered love and helped lift my spirits every time.

When I wasn't online, I would chat with Roisin, who spent endless hours calling and texting me so we both could lift the spirit of one another. As a family, we were big boxing fans. We grew up watching the big hitters such as George Foreman, Mike Tyson, Buster Douglass and Riddick Bowe. We delighted in them ducking and weaving their way through the different belts of the eighties and nineties. Our daughter is named after Muhammad Ali's daughter, Laila Ali, a boxer in her own right, and Lennox after Lennox 'The Lion' Lewis. Growing up, boxing brought us all together as a family. Often our Sunday afternoons were laden with excitement as Dad gave us all the knowledge and information, and we loved the thrill of the fight, especially when we were trying to work out if it was sweat or blood coming from the mouths of the gladiators in the ring. The close of the boxing match guaranteed my sister and me front row seats to a family replay from our brothers battling to be the successor and win the imaginary belt which was usually one of mum's scarves. It was great. I have such fond memories of that time.

My brother, Tony, was born in 1980. Back then, Tony was our new toy, our plaything, and we loved him to bits. When Mum and Dad brought him home, I remember it feeling like Christmas Day. He was our funny little boy and, by the age of eight, he had outgrown both me and Terry. He was, and still is, huge! Standing at six foot four and broad-shouldered, I snugly fit under his armpit. I often wondered what it would feel like to be that tall, to be able to freely reach for things on the top shelves at the supermarket, or to have pole position at a concert without even trying… but as I stand a mere five foot two, I have no chance of that.

Humour is at the forefront of Tony's banter and he carries a sharp wit to be envied. He is a father of four, two boys and two girls, who manage to keep him grounded and on his toes at the same time. He raises money for charity when he can through his gym by competing in boxing matches. He checks in with me and it comforts him knowing that he is part of a larger picture of people who look out for me.

Tony decided to take up boxing just before he turned forty. His newfound fitness saw him winning fights, losing weight and feeling fit. Our family felt proud. How lucky we were to have a man-mountain brother with an equally large heart!

TONY:

I have always been a boxing fan. For the past ten years, I have been committed to training at my local boxing gym. Quite often they would ask me to participate in a boxing match. Not long after Lindsey was diagnosed, I was asked to compete something I had always previously refused. I thought, if my sisters have to fight this cancer battle, then what have I got to worry about? I had six weeks to prepare and decided to make it a charity boxing match with all funds raised going to cancer research U.K. I spent most nights training after work. Before I knew it, it was fight night and I was ready. I was fighting an ex-doorman who had a few wins under his belt and was well-known as a tough guy. Unlicensed boxing is not as glamorous as you would see on the television. It's two hundred people packed into a working man's club, where the longer the night goes on, the louder and rowdier the tightly-packed crowd becomes. I was the last fight of the evening. The main event presented intense pressure.

Roisin never wanted to see me punched in the face so didn't attend, which I can totally understand, although, on the day of the fight, she rang me to give me a pep talk. She told me to imagine that I was punching cancer out of her and Lindsey with every punch I landed. It was the best advice she could have ever given because I knew at that moment I would win, and I did! Third round knockout. It wasn't easy, but it will never compare to Roisin and Lindsey's fight. They are both the toughest of girls. I can only wish to have the strength and bravery they have shown. Even though I don't say it much to them, I love them both so much and I'm very proud of them.

P.S. When John and I fought on Mum and Dad's living room floor in 1993, he caught me with a cheap shot and that was the only reason he won!

During the course of my illness, I was showered with love and gifts. My Homey, Naomi, came over one day, bringing with her some mindfulness adult colouring books, a huge bunch of sunflowers and two Mexican worry dolls for the children. According to legend, children tell their worries to the worry dolls and then place them under their pillow when they go to bed at night. By morning, the dolls have gifted them the wisdom and knowledge to eliminate their worries. I truly loved this. It brought a new spiritual level to my children's night-time routine. We already chatted about what they were grateful for, what had made them smile, sad and happy in their day when we put them to bed, and this was just a needed extra. Just as I could feel my relationship with my children, I could feel my friendship with Naomi strengthening.

A million cuddles with Layla and Lennox were exchanged throughout all of my treatments. I got into the habit of reading to my children. We would bond over various books and it made me feel close to them. Layla, now and again and after some cash-laden bribery, would give me a salon-style manicure and a foot massage. John was the one wrestling on the floor and being goofy while I would shout directions from the sidelines of my chemo chair.

They have coped so very well with what has happened to me. That's not to say it doesn't sometimes creep up on them and frighten them. For example, putting Lennox to bed one night saw him have a really good cry. It was nearly the first anniversary of my mastectomy and only a few days away from his tenth birthday. This must've triggered a memory, which in turn triggered tears. He also played the last recorded message from the love heart speaker inside the Mummy's Wish teddy and went to bed quite solemn. Poor little man. My heart broke that night.

My friend, Vanessa, very kindly organised a system for me that was just lovely. It was called 'Take Them a Meal' which is an online app designed to help out people in times of need. She wrote a pleasant greeting with a welcome and how making a meal was a simple way to contribute, come together and support us as a family, taking the pressure of that evening mealtime. The link was sent through Facebook and, if people wanted to, they simply selected a day and wrote what they would gift us and it took care of itself. I was over-whelmed by her idea and was blessed that this was an option for friends and family. People's generosity astounded me.

HOMEY NAOMI:

'A staff member suggested a meal tree so that there was at least one chore that didn't need to be worried about and the family could continue to eat hearty, nutritious meals. This was graciously taken up by Lindsey, and often I would deliver the meal as I dropped Lennox and Layla home after school – they were lucky that it made it into their house, some of those meals smelled delicious!'

The Otis Foundation www.otisfoundation.org.au specialise in gifting retreat accommodation to those experiencing breast cancer and provide the opportunities for families to relax, reconnect and make memories. The story of our house stay was that unfortunately, a lady named Kerrie Gray died in 2011, aged thirty-eight, leaving behind a magnificent legacy. Situated in a small town in Central Victoria called Redesdale, a stunning, purpose-built family retreat was set on acres of rural farmland. She had a vision and her husband, Paul, through his passion and his building company, partnered with the Otis charity with the result being 'Kez's hideaway'. We were blessed to have the opportunity to stay there.

We arrived on Easter Monday. The roads were quiet and our ute was packed with food, clothes and bikes. The trip was to be lined with both laughter and excitement. 'Wow' is an apt word to describe our home for the next five days. We came through the gates and it was fantastic from the start.

An attractive building boasting a modern, enormous property came into view. The children squealed with excitement!

They wandered around the place choosing their beds, examining the oversized art in detail, and trying to spot kangaroos on the land. Hearing them so excited made a lump appear in my throat. They had experienced a fair bit of trauma over the last year and it was simply lovely to hear pure joy. We read an ode to Kez placed in a frame by the dining table and took time as a family to show gratitude to her. As darkness fell, we spotted a wallaby at our giant glass back doors! More squeals echoed followed by a sprint to film it on the iPad from Layla. I wish she would clean her room that quickly!

The next day was a fishing day. Lennox remarked, 'Not bad for someone who's had cancer', and backed it up with, 'At least cancer gave us a holiday; that's got to be a good thing!' His wit was a sharp as his father's. This trip allowed me to recharge my batteries with my lovely lot after many intense months of different treatments.

It was difficult, but so important to reach out to those who made themselves available to me. I would just have to pick up the phone if I needed a cuppa, a hug, some words of comfort or advice. Being on the receiving end of cards, notes, letters, text messages and skype calls helped fuel me to get better quicker, especially when I was in the hands of the pharmaceutical world. In my situation, the digital warfare was intense, meaning that I was getting so much support via digital means and I'd always feel guilty if I didn't reply. After all, I wasn't working.

Another hot tip: if you know of someone who is going through cancer and you want to help but you don't know how, avoid saying, 'If you need anything, just let me know', or 'If I can help, just let me know.' Why not leave a meal on the doorstep, offer to have their kids for three hours or surprise them by mowing their lawns?

Go to them, call them, take action.

Fifteen

Make some noise

'Everyone hates talking about it, yet everyone knows someone who has died from it. I know it makes people uncomfortable, but I think people need to talk about it more and make it less scary. It's not as frightening as it used to be – having cancer no longer means a death sentence.'
Jake Bailey – cancer survivor

My natural disposition is to be happy. I was raised to meet challenges head-on, but I was also raised to speak up!

Seeing the glass half full is a conscious choice and one I have stuck to most of my life. Playing Polly Parrot by holding repetitive conversations about breast cancer with my family, friends and sometimes strangers could have become tedious, but it didn't; it helped me process what was happening to me, educated them and most of all it allowed me to draw strength from their words of encouragement. Sure there were days where I didn't want to talk about it. I just smiled and said, 'Let's talk about something else', and we would.

While it will never be the end for me and I certainly never wanted this to start in the first place, I wanted to use my experiences to help others. I had the desire to use my leadership and coaching qualities positively. This saw me become the founder of *#checkyourselfTuesday (#CYT)* as it became incredibly important for me to raise awareness about this horrible disease. It took me a while, but it is a thirty-minute presentation on the importance of early breast cancer detection and is supported by BreastScreen Victoria. I carried out my pilot speech to my peers, and I even had a t-shirt, some business cards and a drink bottle made up, which made me feel very professional.

It's important to me to talk to women about breast health to eradicate any negative social ideas. Wanting my experiences to mean something to someone else wasn't for narcissistic reasons in any way; I was just drawn to it. Besides, what else was a girl to do? I wasn't working and I had to engage that foggy brain of mine. I'd found life's groove and began to feel good. One of my personal goals for #CYT was to generate conversation which would promote the 'normalisation' of talking about our 'private parts' socially. I wanted to make talking about it a habit; the more people did it, the easier it might become.

Having good connections with all different types of humans is something I'm good at. Statistics in the field of breast cancer meant that I had every chance of surviving my nightmare, so making a difference in my community mattered. If anything, it would also act as a distraction from the land of irrational thoughts. As the bookings for #CYT gained momentum, my sunflower petals blossomed once more.

Feeling scared, shy or worried when I present at #CYT is foreign to me. I deliver my talks to anyone, anywhere and I'm always looking for the same thing – impact. At the close of one of my early public presentations to a group of ninety women, a lady approached me to say, 'I thought that this was going to just be a boring, sob story about cancer, but it wasn't; you're a natural storyteller, so thank you.' Wow! I was blown away and had bubbles of excitement inside me. They still appear now when I think of that moment. I knew there was something in this. It was a win-win. The audience heard a feel-good story and health tips and I filled my time doing something that made me happy.

A colleague of mine recently pulled me to one side in the school corridor. She wanted to let me know that she thought I was an inspiration and that #CYT worked. To me, this was so rewarding. Triggered by one of my social media alerts and checking herself, she had found a lump. Testing revealed it to be a benign tumour, but without #CYT, she admitted she would never have given breast health a second thought. Checking for her now is a given and she tells anyone who will listen about the importance of checking boobs.

Me – an inspiration no, a foghorn maybe, but I was elated when she said the words, '#CYT works.' It made my day and the teacher in me left her with some homework: she was to lie on her husband's chest and check him for any lumps, sign or symptoms. Men get it too; checking should not just stop with women.

A cancer diagnosis can create such emotional, spiritual and physical weight. Putting myself in the public eye meant that I had to transcend my own needs and suffering, and become the leader I wanted to be. During meetings, opening up to people – often strangers – about my journey leaves me amazed at the short-lived bonds that take place, how deep the conversation can go and, at times, the number of intimacies we share. It feels as if I'm in the right place in my life when I present to an audience – a comfortable place. I want to invite thousands of women to join me to learn how to check themselves. In the future, I want to be more and do more. You only live once, right? It's simple – it just makes me feel good.

A common theme when I'm presenting is that audience members tell me two things. One: they don't have mammograms often enough, or at all, and, two: they don't know *how* to check themselves. I can't stress strongly enough the importance of knowing your body. The way your breasts look *and* feel is your greatest tool to detect change. Investing in that full-length mirror allows the monitoring of not only how your breasts feel, but also how they look. I encourage everyone to have one in their bedroom.

If you do detect something that concerns you, don't google it because this action will almost have you convinced that you have full-blown cancer. Dr Google can be too broad and can lead to feelings of craziness and fear. Take comfort using reputable resources from the amazing organisations that represent us, such as BCNA. Be alert, but not alarmed. Go directly to your G.P. and ask questions; get involved. Never remain idle. Don't be ambivalent about it if you feel there is something different or wrong; just ask for a check. Follow that internal instinct, the gut feeling that whispers to us, and rely on your intuition.

Roisin, before her first diagnosis, was told that it was normal for breasts to change and that it could be milk coming in or even mastitis when she felt her lump. This was reasonable advice, but she did not accept it and pushed for a mammogram because, with a family history of breast cancer and a family to live for, she was not about to take a risk. She held hands with those whispers and pushed. It was a good job really because that 'intuition' led to the discovery of a six-centimetre tumour.

Our Nana Rosaleen, who died of cancer, used to say, 'Don't put off till tomorrow what could've been done today.' Don't be afraid to go to the doctors for a chat, or to build your rapport with them, or to get advice. If you suspect something is wrong, or even find a lump, don't be afraid to get a check; don't procrastinate with the attitude of, 'Oh, it will go away', or 'It's probably my period', and one hundred per cent, **DO NOT** be afraid of results.

A word of advice from me is to stay on top of your breast screening and perform regular breast checks, on Tuesdays of course! Don't be the one who is blindsided by how indiscriminate cancer can be.

February 2019 saw me take part in something that I didn't realise was so big, and I found myself volunteering in a way I never had before. Responding to a late-night message, probably when I couldn't sleep, I replied to Jo saying that I would be available to help out with the BCNA (Breast Cancer Network Australia)/ Bakers Delight campaign in any way. Kellie Curtain, the media manager, contacted me to explain that, along with eight other women and one man, John Thackeray, I would be volunteering to have a photo shoot and to bring along some 'breast friends'. My knee jerk reaction was, *Who do I choose? So many people have supported me – this is going to be hard. To whom do I give the rose?*

Cindy was a given. I had been friends with her not long after immigrating to Australia in 1997. My friend Lauren, who's the most photogenic teacher you could ever meet; Aime and baby Maggie, who I met through our husbands playing soccer together; and Stacey, who's always super supportive to me, were the lucky winners. The photoshoot was held at BCNA head office in Camberwell and we had been warned that it was a campaign with a difference. Some of the photographs would be shot with me wearing a white top and a pink top; in others, I would have on no top at all. However, to remove the nudity aspect, sweet buns and bread rolls would be placed over my particulars. Gulp! I was down for this and ready to have a laugh.

I have never been a wearer of pink, but I rocked it that day. For me, wearing pink for breast cancer displays a sense of solidarity. It brings awareness, helps raise money, makes people feel good about helping others, and is the colour connected directly to breast cancer. It can act as a reminder to us all to breast check and it can act as a colour of remembrance for those who have fought the fight, male or female. Acknowledging that men get breast cancer too is so important, just like when John Thackeray bravely stepped up to represent the 184 men who were going to be diagnosed with breast cancer in 2019.

We were treated with 'make-overs.' Having your hair and make-up done is wonderful. Handing over the responsibility to someone else to make you look glamorous is a feeling I had on our wedding day and before my head-shave. I had the friendliest make-up artist. He looked like he had just stepped off set from *Hawaii Five-0* and had a wild laugh to match. He was brilliant and I looked gorgeous. 'Look Good Feel Better' really was true!

While getting ready, I could hear the giggles of my friends and the excited chatter. Yes, cancer is horrible and life-changing but right then, at that moment, we were forgetting our troubles and stresses and we were having a great time. It left me with a warm, fuzzy feeling. I wasn't nervous at all during that BCNA/Bakers Delight photo shoot and found the whole experience to be a 'delight' (pardon the pun!). We had to tap into our 'brave' on the day – brave because it can take courage to remove some of your clothing, with or without going through a breast cancer diagnosis. The campaign opportunity made some of us step out of our comfort zones and take risks.

It was only at the end of the photoshoot that I learned that there are around 700 Bakers Delights nationwide and that our semi-naked photos would be sprinkled all over Australia! The campaign had a clear message: 'Breast friends' are vital and so important when you are going through a life challenge. Chatting to some of the other survivors on the day was another treat. We had known each other for moments, yet we were quickly sharing experiences and even offering each other advice. It was a fun and unique experience, to say the least.

Cindy: *'It was fabulous and laughing with Lindsey was awesome. I loved the vibe and positivity of everybody involved.'*

Lauren: *'Such a beautiful way to share part of Lindsey's journey. It was liberating to have cancer and laughter in the same room.'*

Aime: *'I loved being part of the "breastie crew", having a laugh about each other's "buns" and having open conversation about breast cancer awareness; just great.'*

Stacey: *'It was a wonderful opportunity to celebrate the strength and vibrancy that day. Lindsey was born to inject others with her infectious spark and this campaign has given all who took part a platform to share their smiles, be noticed and raise donations along the way.'*

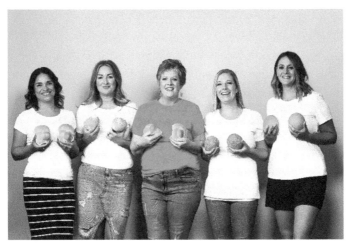

My 'breast friends' L-R: Cindy, Lauren, Myself, Amie and Stacey. Courtesy Nick Blair.

I laughed at the many selfies my family and friends teased me with when they saw me in Bakers Delight stores during the campaign. It simply felt wonderful to be pampered and be part of such an important month. What no one realised was how big this campaign would become!

Two days before the official BCNA and Bakers Delight launch, I was asked to go to Melbourne's iconic Flinders Street Railway Station for a photo shoot. Kellie Curtain (her name is too cool to just write Kellie) and I met with a national newspaper photographer who wanted to capture an image of me in front of an enormous digital poster advertising the campaign. This poster was HUGE and ran around the edges of two buildings. I was both shocked and excited at its enormity.

The poster was in two parts and featured me and two other campaigners, and was positioned at a very busy city junction. The plan was to avoid death at all costs, but capture a good photograph of me in the foreground of the poster. We realised we had eight seconds to nail it, as it was on a loop. Instructed to stand in the middle of the road with my hands on my hips, it was on the third attempt and, without a road traffic accident in sight, we got the shot. It appeared on page five of the national newspaper and I felt a tiny bit famous.

The next day, I met up with Kellie Curtain and Rebecca, another face of the campaign. We were asked to do a short live interview on the morning TV show, *Sunrise*, with Samantha Armytage, one of the hosts of this iconic Australian television show. She vehemently supported the campaign. Reaching the location, I saw two cameramen setting up lights and before we could blink, an ear-piece was thrust our way and we had the producer of *Sunrise* in our ears checking all was in order for a live feed in a few moments. That's when it happened. The nerves kicked in! Anyone who knows me would realise that I qualify for all the following statements: 'Can talk underwater', 'Talk the leg off a chair' and 'She can chew your ear off'. On that occasion, I was the proverbial 'deer in the headlights'. However, I said what I wanted to say about the campaign and left feeling content.

'I believe we have all experienced a very extraordinary scenario from a very unfortunate turn of events for us physically, emotionally and some mentally. Something good has to come from our adversity and, here it is, all of us bonded by a common denominator.'
Nina – BCNA Pink Bun participant 2019

On that same afternoon, I attended the official BCNA and Bakers Delight launch along with the other faces of the campaign. Joint CEOs of Bakers Delight, Elise and David, and the CEO of BCNA, Kirsten, were in attendance, as well as Josh Frydenberg, the Treasurer of Australia. He said he recognised me from the newspaper article and expressed a personal interest in my story. He was kind and warm, and we even made a short video together which finished in us both taking a big bite out of a pink bun together at the end.

Josh Frydenberg, Kirsten and I were asked to give speeches. I was thrilled. I loved that I was asked and felt it was important to represent all of the faces of the campaign. Right before the launch speeches were about to take place, some of us were ushered to one side of the room where Kellie Curtain informed us that Facebook had *banned* the images of us, due to them being 'too rude'. I was astonished and this feeling was echoed by all the other people around me. Early thoughts came from bewilderment and confusion, which soon turned into frustration and anger. In our opinion, Facebook had made a huge mistake and we were about to shout that from the rooftops. The tasteful and respectful images across Australia had to be new, fresh, fun and attention-grabbing to achieve impact and, to hear that Facebook didn't get this, was astounding.

EXCERPT FROM MY SPEECH:

'I know this campaign will impact communities Australia-wide. Money raised is valuable and much needed. Knowing that people of all different demographics will enter their local Bakers Delight, understanding that one hundred per cent of sales from Pink Buns will make

a difference to those who need support from BCNA is heart-warming. This must be very uplifting for the purchaser. You never know who or what is behind each dollar. They might be a cancer survivor them-selves, they might be currently going through treatment, they might be connected to someone who is going through breast cancer and that person is on their mind at the time of purchase, or they might just simply want to help. I know that, in past campaigns, I have always been open to parting with extra money for charity and this year's campaign has been made easy with a fun, happy and thought-pro-voking theme. With that, we all look forward to hearing about people all across Australia doing what they do best and that's tapping into their generosity.'

Following the speeches, we had photos for the media. Those images displayed our genuine upset. We were being robbed by one of the largest social media platforms and wanted to get that message out on a national level. Holding the 'controversial' posters of ourselves in one hand, our thumbs pointing downward mimicking a 'dislike' of Facebook's decision, we heard the cameras click. Disappointingly, they never lifted that ban!

We were generously given a goody bag of keepsakes, which included a poster of us and photographs of ourselves with our breast friends, and I loved it. What treasures! They were going straight to the pool room!

I genuinely thought that was it and that my services would no longer be required. How wrong I was! Over the next few days, it was a media snow-storm. We had seriously caught the attention of the country and overseas, gaining exposure which no one could've envisaged. One morning, driving to work, John heard an inkling of controversy surrounding the topic of our campaign on the radio and he immediately called in. This didn't surprise me. John could always see the other side of the coin. Suddenly my usual routine of getting two children ready for school changed.

He called me moments later. It was around 5:00 a.m. and I was on air in a jiffy. With a croaky voice, underlined with passion for what I believed to be a decision soaked with double standards, I put my opinion across, fully supported by the D.J. This was the best kind of publicity. Kellie Curtain contacted me asking if I was available for more interviews. I was, and this stuff got my adrenalin pumping. Not long after and with our break-fast-munching children in the background, I sat in my pyjamas and did two more live interviews and a podcast. That week went very fast.

Life for me moved on. It was late February and I started entertaining the idea of going back to work. At that point, I had been off for fifteen months and I felt ready. I spoke to my doctors and they agreed that going back to work was a good idea and that I could work full-time if I wanted... but hey, who wants *that*? John pointed out that primary schools were prob-ably not the right place to be, given that I'd just beaten cancer, had had a bacterial infection, my immune system was shot, and most primary school children were 'boob height'.

My wound care nurse, Sue, (who I nicknamed **Sue**perwoman) once said to me, 'If I had a magic wand, you would be the first one I would use it on.' This was a lovely thing to say, but made me realise how dire things had been. By not working, was I going to lose my self-worth? I must admit, this was a regular worry of mine. I liked working, but was cancer going to become my morning, afternoon and night? No way. I needed to use my time wisely.

Enough was enough. During my lengthy pilgrimage, I had lost two friends to cancer, and had two friends diagnosed with breast cancer. Using #CYT, I had to show people that I was not afraid to 'make some noise' by telling people what had happened to me. I began presenting to schools, women's clubs, health centres, footy clubs and my personal favourite, Ballarat Pony Trotting Club, where I shared my story with 360 people on behalf of BCNA. It was also a total buzz to have people use my hashtag #checkyourselfTuesday. Impact – my new favourite word.

> 'Lindsey has a very clear message for us all. Breast cancer, when detected early, has a good chance of being cured, so be vigilant in checking ourselves. Set a reminder in your phone each Tuesday and make time for this simple action. It could save your life. Your children and your family need you.'
> St. Joseph's Primary School, Crib Point, Melbourne

One person who makes himself available for many Australians is actor and the most determined advocate for cancer research, Samuel Johnson. Partnered with his 'Love Your Sister' team, Sam engages community groups with his 'larger-than-life' personality. Lucky enough to meet him, I swapped stories with him about public speaking and we shared a few laughs. To have rubbed shoulders with him made my day. He's a truly inspiring individual and I'm in awe of all the hard work he puts in to try to make a difference in future cancer patients' lives, in particular, personalised medicine to ensure the individual is treated.

> 'Cancer is the last true riddle of our times and we know that it can only be solved with hard science. Despite Federal funding remaining static for a decade, Australia still boasts the best clinical results for breast cancer in the whole world. We are the best with less. Imagine what we could do with more?'
> Samuel Johnson, OAM

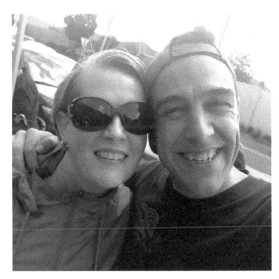

Samuel Johnson and myself in January 2020.
The 'Love Your Sister' team exist to solve
one of the world's most complex problems.

It's my hope that I can encourage people about the importance of breast health. Wishing to change dialogue within families and social circles is important to me; I see it as essential conversation. Why not start now? I challenge you to go and buy a full-length mirror. Go on, make yourself vulnerable – it might just save your life.

I love this short video of Ivy. Take her advice too! Please note where her neck is!!!

For a #checkyourselfTuesday presentation in Australia,
please contact me on: lindseyk262@gmail.com

Sixteen

Life is unpredictable

'What Lindsey has taught me along this journey has changed me as a person and given me a different outlook on life – a better life, one where I will grow old with her and continue to share many memories, dinners, holidays and, most importantly, cups of tea with a side of laughter.'
Martine Carmichael

No finality.
No door-knock to say it's over.
No flowers.
No letter in the mail.
No one to tell you it's over.
It's never the end.

Even though I remain heavily scarred, my scars tell a story of survival. The people in my 'ripple effect' also remain scarred – mine are just visible.

Photographing my journey has allowed me to reflect and process my life with cancer. While it took me some time to be comfortable looking at some of them due to their graphic nature, I truly believe the images have helped support my healing. On the nights I couldn't sleep, I would quietly peruse them and think, *Wow, it was really a rough ride.*

Sometimes, I miss the 'old me'. Sometimes I'm so foggy in my brain, so much that I worry about forgetting details of my life before cancer, I'm afraid I won't be able to recall childhood memories to their fullest, and in weak moments I find this so sad. Cancer, you can take my boobs; just don't steal my past.

Diagnosis, treatment and recovery for me have had many twists and turns! Trying to embrace my new normal and continuing to be courageous is mostly my vibe. Then, that bloody pendulum swings. With its hands around my neck, now and then I feel a little squeeze – just an undesirable reality check from the cancer club! Living with uncertainty, can, at times be difficult. Always feeling like I'm on high alert is tiring, as if I'm waiting for something bad to happen, and then I remember the 'something bad' happened in January 2018. So, here I am in 2020, wondering if I'm cured now. Am I in remission? When exactly do I celebrate my cancerversary? Am I classed as cancer-free? I think I am. I had to ask. I might be cancer-free, but will I be free from cancer, or cancer's threat?

I was desperate for someone, anyone, to say to me that I was done, that all that could be done for me had been and I should consider myself 'fixed'. The truth is it's never really over; it's never the end. Writing that is disheartening.

This intensity surrounding the idea of recurrence can be overwhelming for some of us, but we also understand that cancer may never cash in that return ticket, so we force ourselves to not waste our time, no, *our lives* worrying so much. Through many treatments, Roisin and I have given our bodies the greatest chance to prevent cancer cells growing again, so we needed to allow ourselves to breathe. I know with a strong mindset, solid families and regular checks in order, we *will* reach a point of healthy complacency.

After my lumpectomy surgery, I allowed myself to imagine everyone standing over me cradling bottles of champagne, moving around the room declaring, 'It's gone, it's gone! You're cancer-free', but no. I take the date of my lumpectomy as my date of being cancer-free. The rest is my insurance. So, on 27th February each year, think of me as I toast to living with a chilled glass of bubbles on the back decking, with a happy husband, Layla and Lennox by my side.

I used to hear whispers from long-term survivors of, 'It gets harder after treatment' and I would think, 'No way, not after what I've been through!' But it is undeniably true. After the physical war comes the mental battle. I had to find something to extinguish that – it was time to get my spirituality on. Meditation and yoga have saved me from anxieties about the future. These practices have helped me make peace with the fact that I had the cancerous tumour removed, an infected lymph node taken out, blasted myself with radiation and was made fully toxic with chemotherapy. Every day I draw strength from the fact that both my mastectomy and my oophorectomy pathology were clear! Surely this is enough. What I have learned the most is that the enemy in my head has to remain benign on a daily basis in order for me to move forward.

Physical frailty is often easier to deal with than mental frailty. At times, when I found myself on the perpetual train of worry, I quickly learned to suppress negative thoughts and would place them in the too-hard basket and walk away. How did I silence the voices? How did I find the strength to continually tear the devil off my shoulder? Well, I allowed myself a small window of wallowing, pulled up my fighting pants, and remembered how tough I am. I would rather spend my time being present and enjoying life's moments than allowing scary thoughts to ruin my days. I believed that by doing this, I could keep the bugger at bay.

Life took a turn for the worse, but it carved out a new life for me, and for that, for the most part, I have nothing but gratitude. It would be easy to get down and miserable and have pity parties, but I just made sure I had a few people on speed dial to pull me through my 'wobbly' moments.

At times, 'Hypochondriac' could have been added to my resumé. It is a fine line between being one and not being too dismissive of symptoms. Also, I still suffer pain. Every now and again, sharp, localised electric shock-type pain courses through my eroded left breast. It's pain that is capable of taking my breath away. I hoped it was the nerves trying like hell to reconnect so I would have lovely-shaped, warm breasts that I can feel and that were promised at my initial cosmetic surgery appointment… but sadly re-re-construction is my only choice – that or total removal of the left breast.

Sometimes I imagine what it would look like inside my chest. I'm told the pain is associated with scar tissue. The only way I find relief is to cradle my left breast and push in. It is hard and uncomfortable and aches at the most inappropriate times, such as in the middle of school assemblies!

Another thing I envisage is stepping outside of myself to look at what has happened to me as though it had happened to someone else. *What do you mean you've turned your stomach into breasts and then used your side/flank to rebuild it? Are you joking? That's so weird.* I know that's what I would've thought if someone was telling me that story. Having this surgery changed my physicality, and in turn, my life. It's changed the way I reach for things in the supermarket, the form I take when I stretch, the restrictions I have with gym classes, the way I sleep, the lingerie I buy… so many things are now forever altered.

Our children's lives are also forever changed. They have learned that life is wonderful, but doesn't always turn out the way you want. I love that, even though it has been hard, they have learned a good life lesson out of it. They now know that marching on during difficult times is paramount to a positive outcome.

I honestly believe that if I was a miserable, self-loathing (that could've been easy given the state of my chest) person, who was sad all the time, then managing my cancer diagnosis would have been so much more difficult. Thoughts such as having bad odds, having a bad family history, recurrence, even death, try to penetrate my mind from time to time. When these secret whispers from my subconscious have tried to hang around, I would tell myself, *Sorry I can't talk right now*, and shut them down like an annoying telemarketer and just get right on with what I was doing.

I realise I wasn't informed enough. Watching my nannas, sister and brother go through cancer treatments was one thing, but going through it myself was not what I expected. The aftermath of cancer, what could happen – such as lymphoedema, 'scanxiety', psychological impact, effects of hormone blockers, long-term effects of treatment – were things I knew absolutely nothing about. Call me naïve, but I thought I would have surgery (lumpectomy) and be jumping back in my old shoes and tap-dancing my way through the recovery. Obviously, that didn't happen.

I have learned to really hear people when they talk and to always be 'present' when I'm in the presence of others. When it comes to John, Layla and Lennox, I look at them with more intensity, I stare at them longer, and I stop to look at them instead of juggling the washing while feeding the dog. Being unwell has strengthened my relationships with my family and provided me with a more open heart. I knew I had reached the point now where I had to forget about my collateral damage and move on. The daily demon (am I being dramatic?) was just not welcome anymore.

I will never break my ties with BCNA, BreastScreen Victoria, Think Pink, Breast Intentions, my McGrath Foundation nurses, Mummy's Wish and Camp Quality. These organisations were there for me during my most vulnerable hours. My link with them may lessen, but I know they are there for me always. They were my security blanket for many months and saw me through some really tough days.

One day, I imagined sitting with my doctors as they reported that cancer was back. Even though it was an imagined thought, it made me cry real hot tears. It didn't last long, but while it was there, it was scary and raw. At the time of my real diagnosis, I was cool, calm and collected. This time, I was side-swiping the doctor's desk, like in the movies, and topping it off by using the keyboard to smash the computer monitor.

Waking up these days, I whisper to myself daily, 'Enjoy today and all that it brings.' My senses have heightened, my antennae to life are up and every day is precious in our family. We have to be on guard, sure, but we also have to be adventurous.

I wish for everyone to embrace life. Don't stress in traffic – use it as an excuse to catch up with your favourite playlist and have a car disco; volunteer (one of Layla and Lennox's favourite things to do) because it feels good; do something good for a stranger; have the odd week off social media (okay, by week I mean week… end!); leave a muffin out for the postie; pay for someone's coffee; tell your family you love them more; and sing often. Think of it as free therapy. It is so rewarding to pay it forward.

These days are filled with good things. Each week, I try my best to do something nice for someone. At the petrol station one afternoon, I noticed a man who looked as though my paying for his petrol would be a positive thing. Watching as he made a coffee, I knew this would give me time to pay without him noticing. I approached the cashier and he informed me that the man had two bills – one gas, the other, petrol. Had I set myself up here? Was it going to be in the hundreds of dollars with my bill too? I hadn't worked for eighteen months!! I laughed at the situation. Only I could pick the guy that had two bills! It was no problem. I promptly paid and left with a huge smile on my face.

Attempting to merge with the traffic, I could see the man becoming larger in my rear view mirror. I didn't want to chat. I'd hoped to sneak away before he saw me but I had to stop. When he reached the car, he was a diminutive man with piercing blue eyes and his face told me he'd lived five lives. He was overwhelmed and couldn't stop smiling. He said he'd been down on his luck recently and that he was truly grateful. He asked for my name and I told him 'Lucy', a pseudo name I'd used for years when ordering pizza or Starbucks – easier to spell – and he asked where I lived. I told him that he didn't need to know that information and that he should just graciously accept and have a great day. We shook hands and both went on our way. It felt great… really great.

Life can be fraught with challenges, some bigger than others. It's a cliché, but I try to not 'sweat the small stuff', because the small stuff is exactly that: small and menial compared to the fun there's left to have on this beautiful earth. So, I remove the drama, slow down and enjoy 'the little things'. Cancer is by no means pleasurable, but I have gained pleasurable experiences out of my diagnosis, and some of the new people now in my life are an absolute joy to be around.

One of those people is a nurse named Ange, who once referred to my journey as 'unlucky lucky', which I love. That is exactly right. I am so lucky in so many ways. I just had an unlucky experience. Having to slow down took some adjusting. I was a 'hundred mile an hour' type of person and now I 'breathe life'. I inhale it and respect what it has brought to me. I make time for myself now – something I was really quite bad at. Positivity goes a long way too. I mean, don't get me wrong. We all understood the seriousness of my family situation, but I never once let it bring me to my knees. The eternal optimist in me did not give cancer permission to break me. If it tried to push me around, I pushed back, harder. Mindset can be the biggest weapon against cancer, but it's a choice. Curling up into a ball and crying every day is a choice too, but I chose not to do that, ever.

I also never reached the *Why me?* stage, never. I just remind myself often that I have survived some fairly rough days during my cancer treatment and I have a lot to be grateful for. Tomorrow is not guaranteed for anyone, so enjoy each day. Positivity breeds positivity. There have been times where I wished for my old life back, especially mid-hot flush or catching a glimpse of my chest while changing, but I simply have to get on with living life.

Graduating as a civil celebrant has given me a change of focus and over-whelming love for those people who matter to me. I appreciate 'the little things' more now and it makes me smile. I give thanks for my strength and for the strength I had to not fall apart. People would comment that I'd come through it all so well and always seemed to be smiling. This was followed with, 'Why is that?'. I would satisfy them by admitting it was because I had a good outcome.

Even when I look in the mirror and see remnants of cancer's curse, I never see my cancer diagnosis as death staring me in the face – more that I had to fight to keep it away, a bit like sandbagging. Facing death is not something to which I give much thought.

Cancer is unpredictable. It might try to come back, but for now I rest easy, knowing that we have won our battles. I think of Sean, Roisin and myself and I know that cancer could not, and did not take us down. Having cancer has made me more determined to be a better mum, wife, sister, daughter, aunty and friend all rolled into one. The human body can do amazing things. We witness this when we watch extreme sports – the Olympic Games or cyclists in the Tour de France – but cancer is strong and cunning and a force to be reckoned with.

Cancer did not just affect me; it affected people in my life whom I love deeply. I'm just glad that, on the days I needed it, these people had big shoul-ders for me. Having a good cry is essential; it helps recharge batteries and rebuilds new fight. I suppose the strong woman in me had a fair few days off during my journey, but she never disappeared; she just had some time out. John probably loved the quiet, if I'm honest! I never saw my tears as weak-ness, but as a release of my worries or anxieties that day. I was tested, but I consider myself a much stronger person now. Cancer confronted me and then I confronted cancer. I stared it in the face, but didn't get out unscathed.

So, what is left?

Well, naked, I look like a patchwork quilt. My hair has grown back thicker and healthier, my nails are still paper thin, my sleep patterns are back to normal, but I remain bothered by the very inconsiderate hot flushes.

Feeling strong and determined during my treatments was in my DNA. I had to rely on modern medicine to work to save my life. I took life one day at a time and used friends and family as my safety net. I don't look too far into the future now unless I've booked a holiday and then the children and I do a serious countdown on the whiteboard on my fridge.

I spend my days finding happiness and not looking back, because that is the past and the past has gone. As a family, we take long walks on the beach, stopping to digest the beauty we are surrounded by. We stop to watch gulls overhead, we track aircraft and wonder who is flying them, and wonder where their final destination will be, and I goofy-dance in the kitchen with my children, which I have only recently been able to do because of boob bounce!

Re-evaluating not only my life, but John's, Layla's and Lennox's, has been a natural process. I've embraced spirituality, chat with Roisin most days, try to get outdoors as much as possible, listen to music, surround myself with positive people, use my essential oils, study whenever I can and laugh – a lot. Asking myself what I wanted for the near future rather than the rest of my days has helped me see more clearly. I relish the ability to get up and make breakfast using a pan filled with hot delights, and to sit and eat it slowly, rather than throwing two pieces of bread in the toaster and disappearing to do one of the many jobs I needed to do to get to work on time, often eating that toast on the way. As a family, we embrace new things because now, 'the little things' really are the big things.

Cancer has taught me to live slowly, be present and focus on fulfilling short-term goals, of which I have many. Yes, my stomach and breasts are deformed... but I didn't die. I was challenged by cancer, but I consider myself a much stronger person now.

As breast cancer survivors on opposite sides of the globe, Roisin and I didn't just beat cancer by not dying from it – we survived the copious amounts of testing placed upon us, multiple surgeries and the inside demon that tried to eat away at us emotionally. We determine what happens next and how we craft the rest of our lives through our daily actions.

I know I am not alone when I say that, as a woman, I was unarmed when it came to what I knew behind the scenes about breast cancer. I've learned so much experiencing it firsthand and now I want to continue to help spread the word. There is so much more to it than: 'find a lump, either live or die, the end'.

Roisin is the ultimate cancer kicker. She's lived with the disease for almost six years now and has achieved so much in that time.

ROISIN:

Whilst I still live in daily fear, I really have had an absolutely incredible two years. It hasn't all been tears and vomit. I have written and self-published my first children's book titled, 'Shiny Happy Horace', I was nominated for a BBC Courage Award and raised over 40,000 pounds for Cancer Research U.K., for whom I am an ambassador. After climbing mountains, both physically and mentally, travelling to Australia and America making memories, I'm now a columnist for a U.K.-based national newspaper, The Daily Mirror. I also became a One Show Christmas Angel on the television before finally biting the bullet and leaving my hospital job in order to convert my illness into a business - www.fightypants.com.

The best thing is, I've been alive to feel everything I thought I would miss, such as watching my little Ivy Brown start school and having weekly sleepovers with her. Even kissing my mum and dad on their cheeks when I see them and witnessing the peace on their faces when they know I'm having a good day, is so special to me. Excitedly, we get to plan our 2021 WEDDING! Michael finally asked me after almost eleven years together. Apparently, he doesn't like to rush into things! The best part, after thinking that adoption could never happen, in August last year, we brought home our six-month-old son!

SCREW YOU CANCER.

P.S: I do have to administer lifelong chemotherapy, but as long as I'm here, I really don't care.

Ahh, life! I love you x

I too, now appreciate 'the little things' so much more. I have fairly good health and a functioning body. I am a watcher of my own emotions and I'm aware of how I feel all the time. I have a renewed life now. I have slowed EVERYTHING down and life has now hit a perfect pace. Charities wrapped me up in their arms, my family and friends propped me up, the rest was easy. I don't wish to diminish the severity of breast cancer, rather to suggest, given the right environment, some breast cancers are highly beatable and that social dimensions matter in order to aid healing. I am mentally strong now, emotionally stable and spiritually grounded. I consider myself to be one of Australia's lucky survivors.

As a family, we have been to hell and back, but it's the 'back' that matters. We rise each morning, putting one foot in front of the other, fighting back tears and torment at times as strong, over-qualified warriors. I believe this breast cancer challenge was designed for my sister and me... designed to make us braver, stronger and more appreciative for the rest of our very long lives.

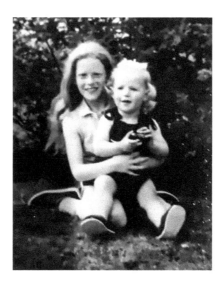

Sisters 1985

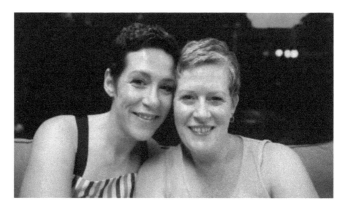

Sisters 2019

Seventeen

The ripple effect

MUM:

'Lindsey has always made myself and her father very proud. Whenever she is up against any form of adversity, she stands and deals with whatever is thrown at her. When she was diagnosed with breast cancer, instinct told me she would do whatever it took to battle for wellness, even against a very rare bacteria that dared to infringe upon her somewhat weakened health.

Late 2018, we decided to join her cancer fight and flew to Australia to support her. It was a very difficult decision because we were placed in somewhat of a predicament as, at the time, both Roisin and Lindsey were mirroring their extensive cancer treatments. Lindsey needed us, and as expected, fresh out of the hospital, and even though incapacitated, she was still good at organising us when we arrived!'

DAD:

'Lindsey called me from Australia to tell me the terrible news. Words can't describe how I felt. She was on the other side of the world, giving me this devastating news and there was nothing I could do except listen. Being the third child of our six children to be diagnosed with cancer left me feeling helpless. Fast forward nine months, my wife and I made the journey to Australia to help care for Lindsey and her family. Whilst John had been her rock, the cold reality of life is that he needed to get back to work, so, for the next three months, we did whatever we could to help out. Lindsey became very ill when we were there. Watching her suffer and spend half the time we were there in the hospital was so hard.

Being beside Lindsey through her illness and watching how she dealt with it strangely comforted me. She has always been my 'determined' daughter. She remained positive, held her sense of humour and, more than anything, kept laughing in her truly infectious way.

I knew Lindsey would kick holes in this diagnosis. We all did. She had too much to live for.'

JOHN:

'I think they found something.'

'Five words that knocked the wind out of me, made me fear for Lindsey's health and feel scared of what lay ahead. When Lindsey called to say that they thought they had found something, I just felt empty. I was in a slight daze and didn't want to think of the negative possibilities.

When it was confirmed as cancer, I immediately went into fight mode. Not flight. Not freeze. FIGHT! What followed were months and months of treatments, illnesses, operations and bacteria. I felt hopeful, but it was marred with gut-wrenching pain and sorrow for the amount of discomfort and suffering the woman I loved was going through.

Lindsey and I spoke so much about beating this disease. Being honest, after Sean and Roisin fought and survived their own cancer, coupled with the family being so strong, I wondered to myself if it was going to be third time 'unlucky' for the third child to be diagnosed. I thought about the life Lindsey had led since leaving England, her family and all her friends. She had travelled, had a career, a home, me, the children and amazing memories. Now she had cancer... was she going to lose it all? Worse still, Layla, Lennox and I were maybe going to lose her.

Our relationship has been one built around communication, love, laughs, travel and adventure. The thought of any of those things being compromised wasn't worth thinking about. Watching Lindsey give birth twice was so inspiring. Accompanying those feelings was the stark realisation that she was so much tougher than I was. That was nothing compared to when I saw first-hand, her resilience and strength throughout all the operations, therapies, meetings, injections and sicknesses.

The Little Things

As a man, father and husband, it was all very tough. Nothing compared to what Lindsey must have felt though. She was the one who woke up each morning wondering about how this evil growth had invaded her body, her life and her family. As a human, it could have been a daily struggle to stay positive, but not for Lindsey. It was with a heavy heart that I went to work every day, not entirely knowing what the next steps would be. To their credit, the specialists were amazing, informed, compassionate and well-planned.

Lindsey not only had me, but also many friends to lean on. I had to show her my strength, push through setbacks and support our beautiful little family. I liked the challenge of supporting Lindsey emotionally and financially. I embraced it. I had no other choice. By lightening the load that Lindsey took on every day with the children and their routines, allowed her to fully concentrate on getting better.

Little things were affected, such as getting out of bed in the morning, school runs, cooking and, of course, making cups of tea. Many of these things were cruelly taken away from her for quite some time.

In the time it has taken Lindsey to return to 'normal', she has completed a course to become a wedding celebrant and has written this book, which has been incredibly cathartic for her. She really is a remarkable woman! She achieved these things whilst undergoing operations, treatments, taking tablets every day and having several hospital stays. She is such a restless person. Sitting still is something she has never been good at, but she had to learn to adjust.

There were many changes to our lives due to the cancer diagnosis. Lindsey's energy levels dropped significantly, as did her ability to stay awake. However, when she was awake and receiving visitors, she was her usual, boisterous self. The issue was that she couldn't keep it up for long and would retreat, exhausted, back to our bedroom once the visitors had left. She loved every visitor that made the effort to visit, drop off food, text, check in with her, deliver care packages and genuinely show interest in her, and us. But I know she hated the fact as to why they were there. We will be forever grateful to every person who showed interest, care, love and compassion. It was unfortunate that those months stretched throughout the year and into the next.

Lindsey is eternally positive. Life is a giant opportunity in which to do something good – great even. She views life as a huge canvas on which to produce a masterpiece. She is a living example of good people doing good things in a bad situation.

Lindsey inspires so many people, but no one more than Layla, Lennox and myself. I have always been good for Lindsey, always seeing the other side of the coin in discussions, sometimes even in arguments too, but she has been a better influence on my life. We complement each other so well. We have been together for twenty-six years with many, many more to go.

The little things in life are the important things.

The important things are the little things that make your life feel fulfilled.

The little things that happen in your life with your loved ones are so personal, so valuable and so special, NO ONE should have to miss out on them. It's the little things that make this world go around and which are paramount to our wellbeing.

'Lins' is the biggest thing in my life, but it's the little things she does with me and the children that make her the best thing in my life.'

LAYLA:

'It was when my dad was working away that I noticed that my mum seemed not to be smiling as much as she usually did. I was ten at the time. The day Mum told me she had cancer was the worst day of my life. She started by saying she had been to get a breast check and that they found a little lump. Immediately, tears welled up in my eyes. Then my throat, stomach and toes stiffened and my hands started sweating. I don't mean a little bit, I mean A LOT. I immediately had visions of men carrying coffins down a church aisle, with my mum inside the coffin. I asked her if she was going to die. To be honest, I was convinced she was going to die, and even when she said she wasn't going to die, I didn't believe her one bit.

She once said that she had a meeting at the bank when really she was getting a breast check. I've since read a few books, and if a parent has cancer, the children of that parent often don't want to tell anyone, but I was the opposite. I wanted to tell.

At school, I wanted only my close friends to know. I know my brother, Lennox, told the whole school, so then everybody knew! We have such a good school. The teachers would come over and let me know if I needed to talk to them, I could. It was nice. Mum started to go to so many appointments. Once she had to go to the hospital every second day and it was an hour's drive away. Sometimes, Lennox and I would have to leave school early. It would be super annoying. She doesn't go to many appointments anymore; it's really good. I know she's getting better, which makes not just me, but us all, very happy again.'

LENNOX:

'I noticed that Mum wasn't laughing that much. She asked a babysitter to look after us while she and Dad just went to the 'bank'; they were going to the doctor to get a check-up on her boobs. The day she told me that she had breast cancer was the day that my dad was in Queensland for work.

Mum video-called Dad and my day had been going perfectly. After school, my cousins were coming over for a play. Mum told us the terrible news – that she had been told she had cancer! She said it was only a bit of cancer and that it was really small. Straight away, I felt heartbroken. Then I asked for the chocolate I saw on her bedside table. "Are those smarties for us?" "Yes," Mum said and she let me have them. They were from Martine, one of my mum's many friends. That's why she had not been smiling much. I knew something was up. When mum told me the terrible news, I thought to myself: What if she dies? She told me that there was a very high chance of her NOT dying. Then I calmed down a bit.

Mum is much better now. She is going to the gym and we even have dance-offs in the kitchen. She is the biggest inspiration in my life *because she climbed a mountain in the Cook Islands not too long after an operation!'*

ROISIN:

'Incredibly, a fundraiser was set up for "that airport hug" and in December 2018, WE GOT THE HUGGGGGGG. Oh my GOD! It was the absolute best hug in the whole universe. We touched each other's faces and hair and cried. She hadn't known I was coming. I LOVE SURPRISES!

We spent Christmas all together with our parents and children and, although Lindsey was still really unwell, it was so special and it gave us that boost we both needed to crack on with treatment once we had to leave each other.

Lindsey will attend our wedding soon, to be my most cherished maid of honour, and I know on my special day, it'll be even more extra wonderful to have my big, healthy sister by my side.'

(Unfortunately, at the time of publishing this book, the world has gone into lockdown mode because of the COVID-19 virus spread, meaning that this trip won't be taking place after all. Another challenge but one that won't break our spirits or our sense of solidarity as a family.)

SEAN:

'A feeling of complete uselessness overwhelmed me when my sister, Roisin, was first diagnosed with cancer. I wished cancer upon myself again. I cried from the pit of my heart. Not being able to take away her pain hurt so much. Luckily her daughter, Ivy, was born early and completely healthy, and this gave Roisin something to fight for. She fought hard and has gone on to become a great advocate for cancer awareness. After only a short time, her cancer returned. I can't even imagine how my sister, Lindsey, felt being so far away from her little sister. Lindsey has lived in Australia since 1997 and I can assure you the news that was coming wasn't a "good day, mate". After trying to *digest the discovery of Roisin's relapse, Lindsey took to Facebook to post an awareness message, warning females to check themselves and proceeded to inform people that she would be going for a screening.*

What we thought was a positive message, incredibly, turned into a more devastating discovery. When I found out that my Lindsey, living on the other side of the world was diagnosed with cancer, I was heartbroken. Even though I knew she was incredibly strong by nature, had an amazing husband and two of the best kids I've ever met, she was still on the other side of the world. I couldn't give her a big hug. It was devastating for everyone, especially me, because Lindsey was living in the U.K. when I was diagnosed, and John's and her love helped me through my journey. I knew she could beat it and she did. Although we've experienced turbulence and the oxygen masks have been ejected more than once, the clouds are certainly clearing for us, allowing us to now be the best versions of ourselves.'

TERRY:

'They say being the oldest is a tough job.

By the time Sean was diagnosed with non-Hodgkin lymphoma, I wasn't living at home and didn't understand or see the impact of how it devastated my parents, brothers and sisters. My youngest brother was seriously ill from a type of cancer that I didn't know anything about and I was quite ignorant of the whole thing. Honestly, back then I was more frustrated that Mum and Dad bought him new D.J. decks, records and everything he wanted – what an absolute shit I was! I was managing this all wrong!

We all thought we were done with cancer, but later, we found out about Roisin's double diagnoses. How could this happen to another family member again? The whole family was devastated, I mean completely devastated. Roisin is such a caring person, an absolute shining star on the world and the glue that keeps our family unit together. I have never seen a person go from racing through life at a million miles per hour, loving absolutely everyone and everything, to instantaneously stopping. She wasn't bothered about herself; she only cared that Ivy might grow up without a mum and Michael would grow old without a wife.

This is where our story took a turn for the worse. Lindsey's results were also positive. How the Holy Fuck can this happen? Why was life being so unfair? Both Roisin and Lindsey had lived healthy, active lifestyles. They didn't smoke or over-consume alcohol (unfortunately, I did) and they had fairly clean diets. How is it that two wonderful human beings who treat their bodies right and look after themselves with such integrity get this horrid fucking disease, yet someone like me who, until recently, didn't care what he smoked, ate or drank got nothing? I felt helpless. I thought, there's nothing I could do to help, apart from offer emotional support. I think it broke me a little.

Thankfully, now Roisin and Lindsey have kicked cancer's ass. Unfortunately, some complications may last a lifetime, but they both still smile every day. I decided that enough was enough. My family have been through enough pain and suffering than anyone ever should endure, and, with my lifestyle, you can bet it wasn't going to be long before I fell victim to some form of illness. I guess you could say I felt like a sitting duck. I joined a gym, The Transform Hub, the very next day. They have helped to transform my life.

I owe my two sisters an overwhelming amount of gratitude for giving me the push to better myself. I adore the strength of my family. Both Roisin and Lindsey are an inspiration, not just because they beat cancer, but because of HOW they beat it. I am so proud to be their brother. Can I still claim that being the oldest is the toughest? Naaah, not a chance. I've had it easy compared to Sean, Roisin and Lindsey. These guys are the stuff that tough is made of.'

TONY:

'When my youngest brother Sean, the baby of the family, was diagnosed with cancer as a teenager, it was devastating for all the family. He fought cancer and beat it. Some years later, lightning struck twice and my youngest sister, Roisin, was diagnosed with cancer whilst pregnant. She too fought it and beat it. Unfortunately, that bastard *reared its ugly head once more and Roisin had a second diagnosis. As a precaution, Lindsey went for a check-up and, unbelievably, at the same time, was also diagnosed. It was a very frustrating time and impossible for me to understand just what they were going through. I often thought to myself how this disease had struck the three of my siblings who I would consider led healthy lifestyles. It just didn't seem fair, but I knew if anyone could grab it by the scruff of the neck and beat it, it would be our Ginge!*

In 1991, Lindsey and I were in Belfast visiting our grandparents. She took me to the cinema to see 'The Commitments'. A small group in the seats behind us began throwing coins at my head. Just before I had time to feel scared, Lindsey stood up and gave them an almighty bollocking and the coin throwing stopped. I was so surprised, but also very proud! She's the type of person who will stand up for her rights and never be afraid to air her views. I respect that. We are a close family, and knowing that she was the other side of the world from us, was so frustrating. Knowing she has a good guy in John brings me comfort.'

MICHAEL:

'It is horrible being the brother of three siblings who were diagnosed with the nasty arsehole of a disease called cancer. I was young when my brother fought for his life and that was the hardest time of my life. To be with someone every day and then to see them so gaunt and ill broke my heart. I was young too, and not knowing how to handle this or what to say to him, sent me off the rails a little. But maybe this was my practice run as I believe that experience helped me later in life, when both Roisin and Lindsey were struck by this horrible disease that is relentless.

It is so frustrating seeing someone you love hurting and worrying and not being able to take the pain away. I would have taken it from them in a heartbeat if I could. To learn of Lindsey being diagnosed while on the other side of the world hit me hard. This couldn't be real – three siblings out of six. It was something you read about in magazines.

Lindsey to be on the other side of the world from us all was tough. I couldn't imagine how she could tell her children her diagnosis. When a child hears the word "cancer", they almost instantly think death. It must have been horrible.

I have three amazing children who are my world and, if I had to ever tell them this, I'm sure it would break their hearts and mine. I can't imagine the heartbreak the kids were going through. They were so young at the time. I know how hard it was for Roisin to have that difficult conversation with daughter, Ivy. She couldn't move from bed for over a week, crying and torturing herself. How could Lindsey do this as well? I didn't know what to say that could possibly help. I will be seeing Lindsey soon – the first time since she was diagnosed – and I can't wait to give her a huge cuddle and for our kids to play together. I now appreciate how strong my siblings are at kicking cancer's arse!'

CINDY:

'The life-changing phone call from my dear friend, Lindsey, informing me of her breast cancer diagnosis felt surreal. Our long friendship is based on pleasurable times spent together – crying whilst watching chick flicks, sharing embarrassing body secrets and 'Tena Lady' moments induced by laughing. Both my mother and grandmother had lived and survived through breast cancer. Their struggles with the disease had deeply affected me and was a dark, looming cloud over my health, especially since I was a mother of two daughters. I screamed when she told me, and punched the wall before sobbing into my husband's arms.

It has been a while since Lindsey's diagnosis and I have tried to be a supportive friend, phoning her most days to check in, holding her hand when she needed it, and trying to act normal in an abnormal situation. Lindsey has shown enormous mental strength and courage throughout the whole journey. She has faced many obstacles in her recovery. At many times, it has seemed that she was taking one step forward and two steps back.

Twenty years ago, I chose Lindsey to be one of my best friends because we share the same family values and zest for life. Lindsey has not changed. Breast cancer has not won – it has made her more lovable, positive and kind-hearted. Today, I love and admire Lindsey more than ever. She has flipped a negative situation and experience into a life lesson, which she now actively shares with others.'

HOMEY NAOMI:

'One sunny day in January, I answered, as I usually did when Lindsey phoned, pretending to be a sexy call girl! Lindsey's reply was flat. She'd had a routine ultrasound and a lump had been found. I was outside playing with my kids, so I hid around the side of the house to mask my worry and tears. Lindsey was so brave, telling me everything was going to be ok. It was only a small lump and she was required to have a needle biopsy as soon as possible. I swallowed hard when she told me there was no way she could tell Roisin or her parents – how could she? They were fighting their own battle over there. So I pulled my big-girl knickers up, told her that no matter what was to happen, I would be there every step of the way and help John and the kids as best I could.

On the first day of the 2018 school year, I fought back tears as our principal informed everyone of Lindsey's diagnosis. Everyone's shock was a ripple that could be felt as the worry swept over us. But, just as quickly, and as good Catholic teachers, we prayed for her, then made a joke, then made plans to support the Kennedy family. She was finally well enough to return to work as a casual relief teacher and everyone, staff and students, were really glad she was back. But nobody was as happy as me!'

SHELLEY:

'When I first heard the diagnosis I was devastated for Lindsey, John and the kids. I just couldn't believe that this horrible disease had encroached on one of the sunniest and loveliest people I knew, especially after all those years of her convincing me that cancer would

never get her. I decided to make this difficult journey a little easier for her by being there whenever I could. I was ready to be by her side as she took on this battle. Even through such a taxing time, she still had her kick-arse sass. One particular day saw her stand up to a nurse who was grumpy and being quite rude. She took on the cancer fight with strength and a good sense of humour like I knew she would. Even when the journey took many detours, she took it all in her stride and not once did I hear complaining. To me, she is an amazing tower of strength and inspiration.

Seeing her was the highlight of my week. Making a meal may have helped, but those weekly visits gave me so much more. It hurt me seeing Lindsey in pain, having to go through chemo, radiation and endless surgeries. It is still something I need to process. It's physically painful seeing someone you love struggle. However, I believe it brought us closer. Lindsey is someone I admire and love dearly and, lucky for me, she's stuck with me for life.'

MARTINE:

'From the moment I met Lindsey, I knew she would be a special part of my life. I didn't realise then how close we would become and how much our families would mean to each other. Our relationship flourished when Lindsey and John moved onto our street just before they got married. Our years were filled with BBQs, pool days, lots of laughs and fun times. I remember when beautiful Layla was born and not long after our 'surprise' package called Olivia arrived and to this day our daughters have a special friendship, just like their mums.

Lindsey called me one night to say that she had been diagnosed with cancer. This news shattered me and my family. Why? It's so unfair, *was my first thought, but another part of me immediately thought,* Lindsey is so tough, one of the strongest women I know, and if anyone can beat this, she can. *So her journey began. I was astonished at how many appointments Lindsey had to attend and I wanted to do everything I could for her. Even though I had a very busy life working, going to the gym and having three children, I knew that I needed, and wanted, to give Lindsey as much as I could in the form of an 'ear'. I would regularly drop in for a cuppa, choosing a tea bag from her very extensive range of teas. Often I only had thirty minutes to an hour to spare, but we would always chat non-stop, allowing me to catch up on her progress, and more importantly, share a laugh.*

Most days saw Lindsey upbeat and positive, but I remember one day, Lindsey answered the door in tears. Even the strongest and hardest have their down days. By the time I left, I'd managed to cheer her up and Lindsey had a smile back on her dial. Laughter really is the best medicine. She continues to inspire me every day with her passion and her work for early detection. Even when the chips are down she continues to give to others. The road ahead may be rocky, but I will always be by the side of this amazing human.'

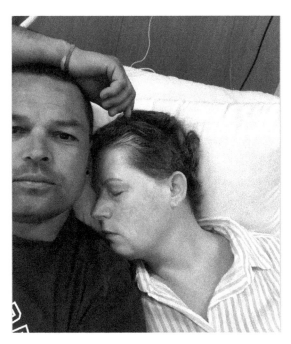

Everyday I am with you, I witness your sheer strength and pure love. Thank you John.

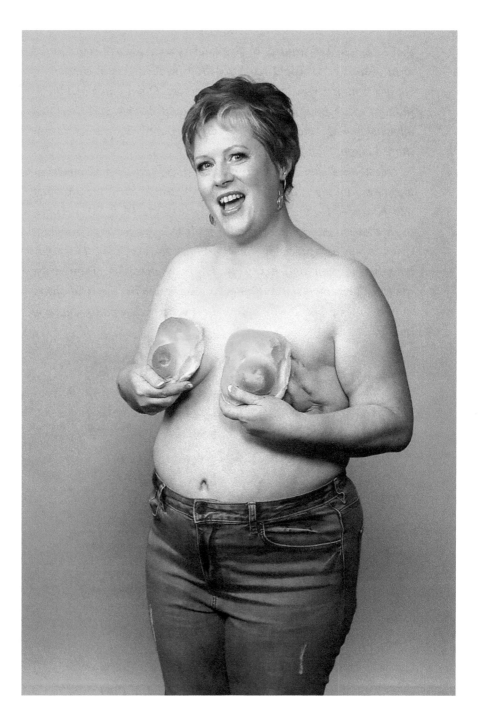

Photo courtesy of Nick Blair

*Along this journey, you need to be able to feel like you can ask any member of your care team **ANY** question.*

SUGGESTED QUESTIONS TO ASK AT THE TIME OF DIAGNOSIS
- What type of cancer do I have?
- What stage am I? What determines this?
- What grade (aggressiveness of the tumour) is it?
- How do you decide what treatment I will need?
- What kind of treatment will I need? What will that look like?
- Do I need more tests?
- How long will I need off work?
- Can I have a copy of any results/paperwork for my personal records?
- Can I do genetic testing?
- Has the cancer spread anywhere else? If so, how can you tell?
- What costs should I expect?
- Can you refer me to a support group/counsellor or any way I could better inform myself?

QUESTIONS TO ASK BEFORE LUMPECTOMY
- Will my current medication interfere with anything that you do?
- From what time should I not eat or drink?
- How long will my hospital stay be?
- How much of my breast will be removed?
- What will the scar look like?
- What size scar should I expect?
- Is there a chance I may wake up with a scar that I wasn't expecting?
- What standard size margins do you take if the tumour looks different once the breast surgery is underway?
- How will you know if it is all gone?
- Will I be allowed to wear underwire bras in the future?
- What is the recovery time/ how long does it take to heal from a lumpectomy?

QUESTIONS FOR INITIAL CONSULTATION – ONCOLOGY
- How do you select the chemotherapy I will be having?
- How long does each treatment go for?
- Do I have to stay in hospital?
- Can you be allergic?
- What if I have an allergic reaction to it? What then?
- Will I still be able to work?
- Will I definitely lose my hair?
- How long will it take to fall out?
- Will my appetite/weight change?
- Are my chances of recurrence high?
- How long will I be monitored after the cancer removal?

QUESTIONS – RADIATION
- Where will you radiate me?
- Does the machine touch you?
- How will you know that you are not damaging my healthy tissue?
- What side effects can happen?
- Will I have side effects such as pain or discomfort afterwards or burning?
- I need to work full-time. How will I fit it in?
- How can I manage side effects if I experience them?
- Can I lift things during treatment?
- If things go wrong and I need help or support, who do I call?
- How long is recovery?
- How might I feel at the end of my radiation?
- Can I wear deodorant or moisturiser as normal?
- How long is radiation in my system?

QUESTIONS – DOUBLE MASTECTOMY

- What will my scars look like?
- How long will I be in the hospital?
- Will I be in intensive care for any of that time?
- How will my pain be managed?
- Where will my drains be?
- Tell me about the risks.
- How long will my surgery take?
- How long until I return to work?
- How long before I can drive?
- How long before I can exercise?
- How long do you recommend I have off the gym?
- How many phases (surgeries) will I need?
- What are some common complications with this type of surgery?
- Will I see you post-op to tell me how it all went?
- Do you have any pictures of the scars?
- Where will I be numb? Will it be permanent?

QUESTIONS BEFORE OOPHERECTOMY SURGERY

- Can I take my medicine as normal on the day of the procedure?
- Can I use lotions, creams and perfume as normal before the procedure?
- How long will it take for my periods to stop?
- What side effects can I expect after this surgery?
- Will I experience menopausal symptoms straight away?
- If I want children in the future, is this possible? (This question refers to fertility preservation.)
- How long is the recovery?
- How long before I can drive?
- How long before I can resume my gym membership/exercise?
- Will I have dissolvable stitches or ones that require removal?
- How long will the procedure take?
- When can I go home?

QUESTIONS FOR INITIAL COSMETIC SURGEON MEETING
- Is the procedure you have in mind my only option?
- What is the rate of success with a procedure like this?
- How long does the procedure take?
- Could the procedure fail?
- Is there anything in particular I should do before going ahead?
- Can I see some before and after shots?
- How many of these procedures have you performed?
- Will I lose sensation?
- Can I keep my nipples?
- How many D.I.E.P. surgeries have you done?

Notes

Notes

Notes

Notes

Notes